Mindful Based Healing

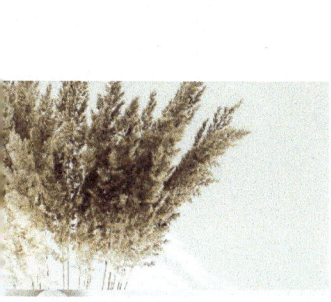
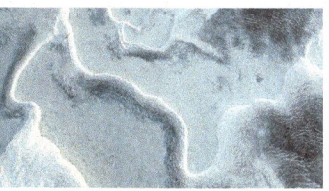
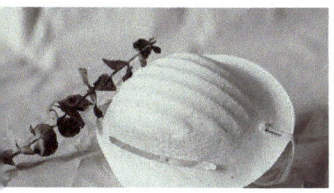
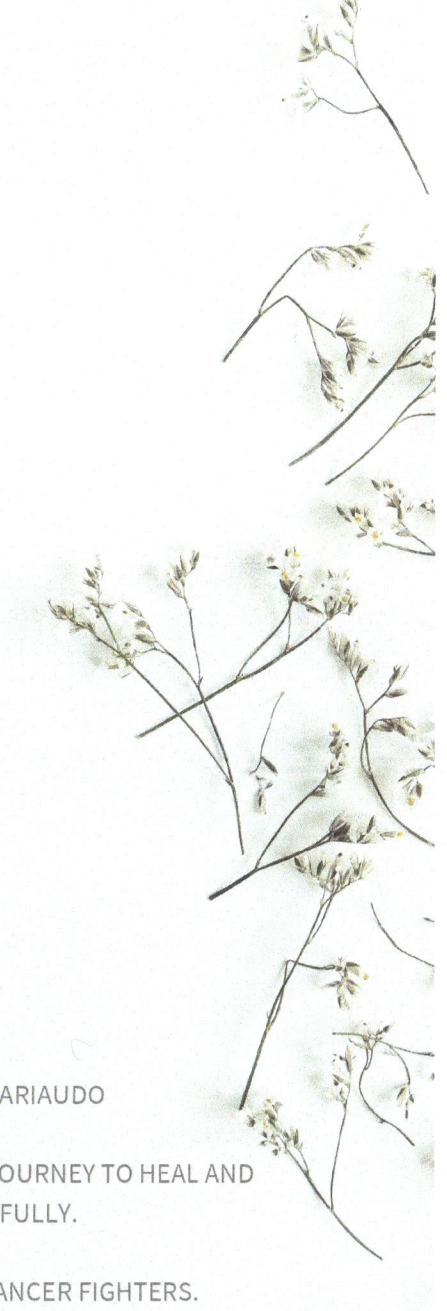

WRITTEN BY: SARAH ARIAUDO

DEDICATED TO ANYONE ON THE JOURNEY TO HEAL AND ENJOY LIFE MORE FULLY.

A SPECIAL DEDICATION TO CANCER FIGHTERS.

To get the most from this guidebook, visit:
MindfulBasedHealing.com/courses

COPYRIGHT ©2021. SARAH ARIAUDO, MINDFUL BASED HEALING, LLC.
All Rights Reserved. No portion of this book or content may be reproduced, transmitted or stored in any form or by any means, electronic or mechanical, including photocopying, recording, or by any information storage and retrieval system without explicit permission in writing from the publisher.
Published by SARAH ARIAUDO/PRINTED AT LULU.COM
ISBN 978-1-304-80433-4

WWW.MINDFULBASEDHEALING.COM

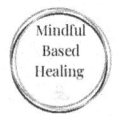

This guidebook is supporting the healing journey of:

beginning on:

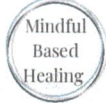

SARAH ARIAUDO
MEET THE AUTHOR

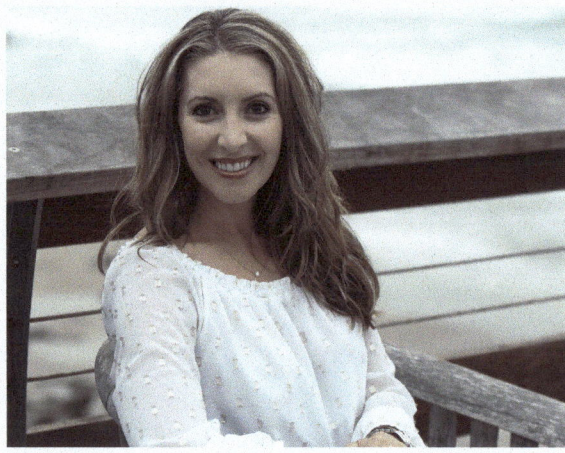

Hi! I'm Sarah,

Founder of Mindful Based Healing. I've worked with cancer fighters since the early 2000s. I've treated thousands of people with Radiation, taught Yoga for Cancer Recovery, managed multiple treatment centers, and helped hundreds of cancer centers to be more efficient in their treatment process. Over the past 20 years I've noticed a trend.... the people who tolerated their treatment the best, healed the quickest, and those who were overall healthier mentally and physically, had a mindfulness practice.

I've also used mindfulness in my own healing journey since 2007. From unexplained health issues, exploratory surgeries, multiple miscarriages, to C-section surgery and recovery; I have used mindfulness techniques to cope and heal through it all. Once I started prioritizing myself and my health, I realized what's important to me. I began to implement the right tools, and as a result, I improved my health, mindset and quality of life. I wish for you the hope, health and healing you deserve. It's time to *thrive*, not just *survive*.

Please know there is no "right" or "wrong" way to do this program. Show up, give it a try, that is success.

'What lies behind us and what lies before us are tiny matters compared to what lies within us'. -Ralph Waldo Emerson

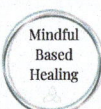

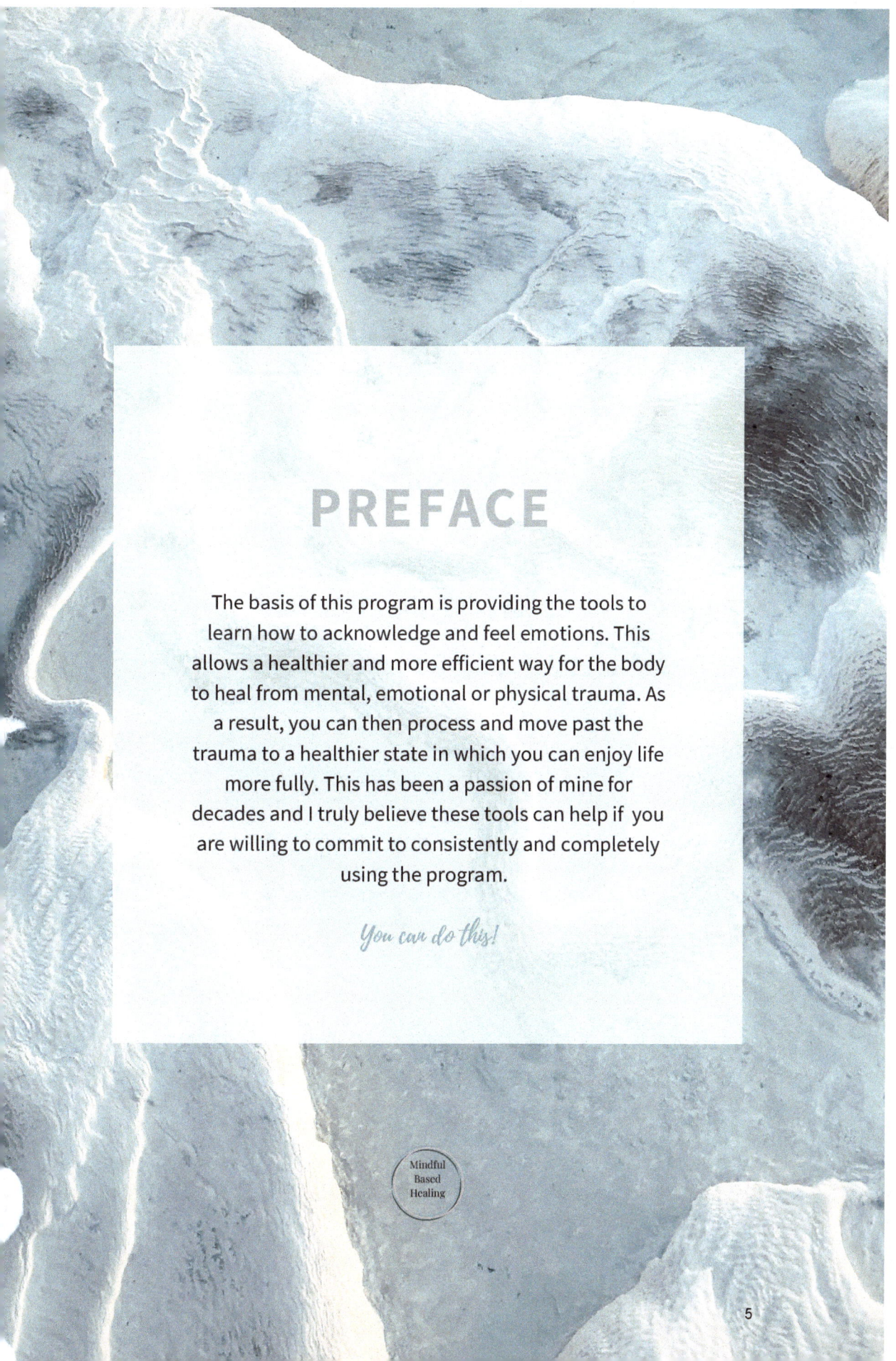

PREFACE

The basis of this program is providing the tools to learn how to acknowledge and feel emotions. This allows a healthier and more efficient way for the body to heal from mental, emotional or physical trauma. As a result, you can then process and move past the trauma to a healthier state in which you can enjoy life more fully. This has been a passion of mine for decades and I truly believe these tools can help if you are willing to commit to consistently and completely using the program.

You can do this!

Mindful Based Healing

For friends and family:

Support for the healing journey

People don't like to ask for help. Use these ideas to support your loved one.

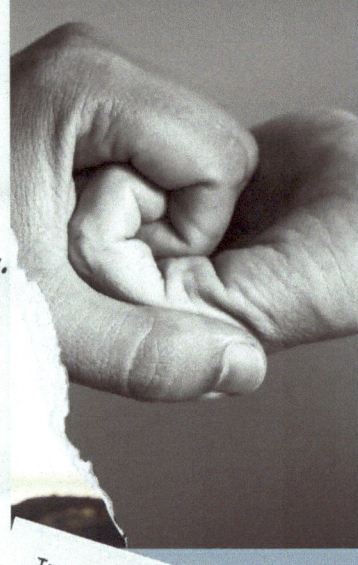

 Coordinate care-Be the leader in friends and family taking turns to help, give updates, make calls.

 Drive- Take your loved one to and from appointments, pick up medication, etc.

 Food- Cook or drop off food to fuel your loved one

 Pets or kids- Feed the pets, walk or play with them. Watch the kids. Your loved one may not have energy and need a nap

 Clean- Clean the house, run errands, fold some laundry. Tidy up to provide a clutter free environment for your loved one to rest, heal and thrive.

Instead of: "Let me know if you need anything" ask: "Do you want me to bring food or have it delivered?" "Do you want me to take care of kids/pets tonight or tomorrow?" "Which appointments can I drive you to?"

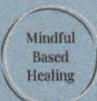

"The only thing that is ultimately real about your journey is the step that you are taking at this moment. That's all there ever is."
- Eckhart Tolle

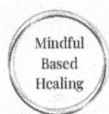

THE PLEDGE

"The only way to live is by accepting each minute as an unrepeatable miracle."
- Tara Brach

I, _____, believe I am worthy of committing fully to prioritizing my mental, emotional and physical well-being. I am actively and independently deciding that on this day, _____, 20___, I am open to experiencing the benefits of this program. I am open to learning techniques that support me in my healing journey. I am open to learning how to be my own advocate, to empower myself to speak up and assist my healthcare providers by more effectively communicating my needs and how I am tolerating treatment. I am creating a new version of me which supports me in being present and enjoying my life more fully.

I commit to learning openly and fully how to be present and aware in my body. I commit to exploring my patterns and coping mechanisms. I commit to choosing a life that supports my healing and holds true to my values and priorities.

I will be an active participant in my health, recovery and life.

I commit to practicing loving-kindness to myself and others. I commit to giving myself grace. If I miss opportunities to prioritize my well-being, I commit to refocus and make choices that support me. I commit to not pressuring or judging myself, but rather challenge myself to be my best version possible at the present moment. I recognize that joy is in the moments, not the minutes and agree, to the best of my ability, to fully commit to enjoying my life.

_____ _____
Signature   Date

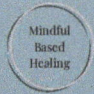

CONTENTS

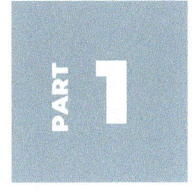

CANCER DIAGNOSIS, NOW WHAT?
Tools to support you in navigating your diagnosis and appointments throughout your healing journey.
- Treatment options, questions for providers, resources for support

INTRODUCTION TO MINDFULNESS AND BREATHING
What is mindfulness and how it can support you.
- Mindful breathing: balanced, belly, box, 2x, cleansing Body scan

MINDFULNESS AND BODY AWARENESS
Mindful body exercises
- mindful eating, mindful walking, mindful movement

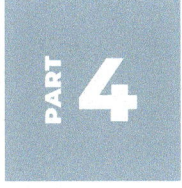

TYPES OF STRESS AND EFFECT ON HEALTH
Learn different types of stress:
- Mental, emotional and physical stress
- How stress effects overall health and well-being

PATTERNS, BARRIERS AND COPING
Learn key concepts and coping techniques to be more present.
- Understand emotions, coping mechanisms, and patterns
- Coping techniques for awareness: 3Ps, STOP, RAIN

CONTENTS

POWER OF POSITIVE THINKING
Self-care and self-talk can have a great impact on healing. Learn tools to facilitate a positive mindset to best support healing:
- Loving-kindness to others and self
- Mindful listening and talking

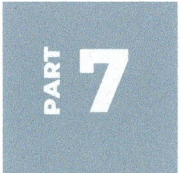

MINDFUL COPING WITH SYMPTOMS AND EFFECTS OF TREATMENT
Learn how to cope with cancer related symptoms and side effects:
- pain, fatigue, body changes, new identity

MEDITATION STYLES
Research has proven the benefits of a meditation practice. There are various types of meditation. Learn and find the technique(s) that work for you:
- Meditation styles: Focused, mantra, guided, loving-kindness

BEYOND TREATMENT, FINDING YOUR NEW NORMAL
Tips to navigate your new normal.
- Priorities, self-care, work/life balance
- Daily mindfulness

INSPIRATION AND RESOURCES
Music, art and reading can help you find strength and inspiration
- Song list and book recommendations
- Reference list for a deeper dive

SELF ASSESSMENT
PRE-MINDFUL BASED HEALING

TODAY'S DATE

CATEGORIES

Please scale the following from 1-5
1 being excellent, 5 being poor.

Excellent-1   2   3   4   Poor-5

How would you rate your overall health?

How well have you been sleeping?

How is your mental and emotional health?

How is your anxiety level?

How is your current ability to cope with pain?

How much do you fully enjoy life?

Do you currently have a Mindfulness practice?

Yes   No   Unsure

NOTES

SCALE

1 = Excellent

2 = Very good

3 = Acceptable

4 = Having difficulty

5 = Poor

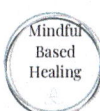

COURSE PROMISE

No matter where you are in your healing journey, this guide will support you. This program was created to teach you the foundation of Mindfulness, with guided exercises tailored to teaching you awareness, breathing techniques and better coping mechanisms that will support you in life.

The tools in this guide are based on over 40 years of scientific research, inspired by the works of John Kabat-Zinn at the University of Massachusetts for Mindful Based Stress Reduction, various methods of mindfulness exercises, meditation, and yoga as well as key concepts from various leadership trainings. I have curated the most accessible and universal techniques to enable anyone, anywhere to benefit. Grounded in research, this program is not founded upon or affiliated with any religious or ethnic group; instead, it is meant for anyone looking to be happier, healthier and more present in life.

You will get what you put in. With consistency, you will be more aware of thoughts, patterns, and coping mechanisms. You will be more aware of your body and how it feels. You will have the ability to be your own advocate and help your healthcare provider give you the best care and treatment available. Learn to speak up, have difficult conversations, ask for help, prioritize your health and well-being.

You deserve to thrive, not just survive.

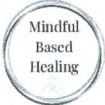

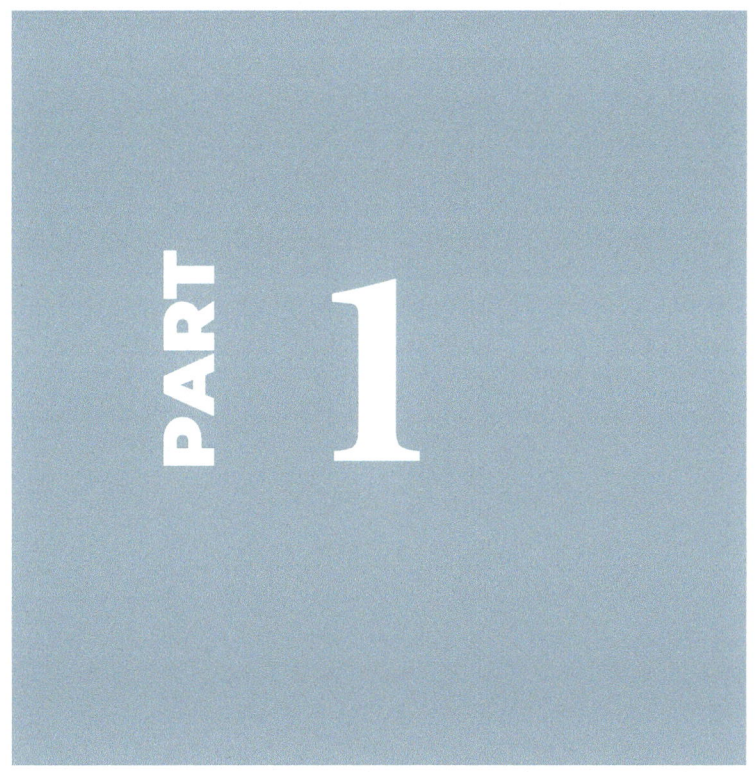

CANCER DIAGNOSIS, NOW WHAT?

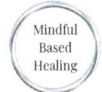

Beginners Mind

"In the beginners mind there are many possibilities, in the experts there's only one". Be willing to see many possibilities. Start with ordinary situations or people you know. Are you truly seeing and experiencing them or do you have pre-conceived expectations from past experience or interaction?

YOUR JOURNEY

You are embarking on a very personal journey. Regardless of how many family members or friends are with you, no one truly understands the emotions, thoughts, or physical sensations you are experiencing. It's not their fault. It's not your fault. Regardless of "why" you are here, this is now your path. Keep putting one foot in front of the other, breathe, and try to be present in the current moment. You can do this!

ASK FOR HELP

Asking for help is brave, not weak. It's empowering, both for you and for your support team. People want to help but don't often know how. Speak up for yourself. Listen to your inner awareness and support yourself by using the resources you have or asking for additional help. Be brave, you deserve it.

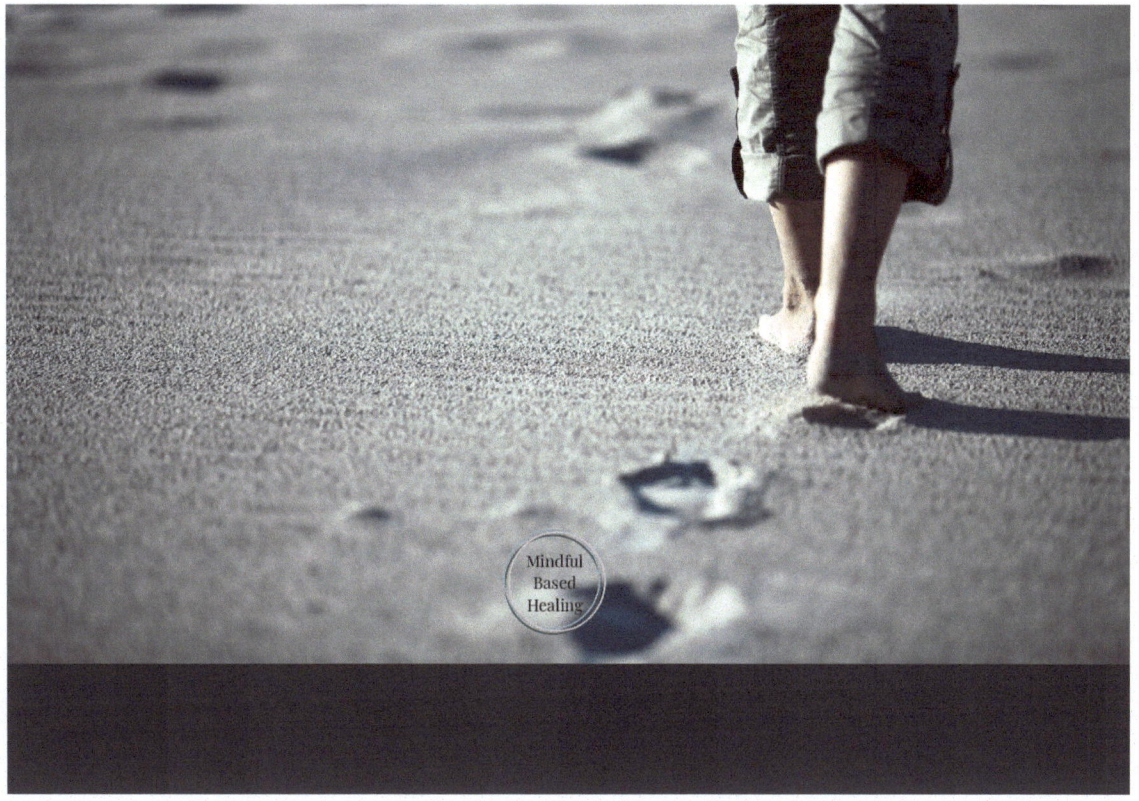

WHAT CANCER CANNOT DO

Cancer is so limited...

It cannot cripple love.
It cannot shatter hope.
It cannot corrode faith.
It cannot destroy peace.
It cannot crush confidence.
It cannot kill friendship.
It cannot suppress memories.
It cannot silence courage.
It cannot steal eternal life.
It cannot conquer the spirit.

— Author unknown

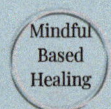

HEALING JOURNEY

"If you aren't in the moment, you are either looking forward to uncertainty, or back to pain and regret."
- Jim Carrey

Welcome to your healing journey. Whether recovering from surgery, still processing a new diagnosis, undergoing chemo or radiation therapy, or struggling with *what now*; please know, you are stronger than you think. This guidebook was created to help facilitate and guide you on your healing journey.

I encourage you to shift from "what is happening *to* me", to, "what opportunity is this providing *for* me."

You deserve to *thrive*, not just *survive*. You will learn what mindfulness is, how it can support you in healing and in life. No one is guaranteed tomorrow. Power lies is enjoying *now*.

"Few of us ever live in the present. We are forever anticipating what is to come or remembering what has gone."
- Louis L'Amour

Mindfulness is experiential, which means you will receive from this guidebook and course what you give. Be open to learning, experiencing, and bettering your life. Take the pledge. Prioritize your mental, emotional and physical well-being.
You deserve it.

"Today, you can decide to walk in freedom. You can choose to walk differently. You can walk as a free person, enjoying every step."
- Thich Nhat Hanh

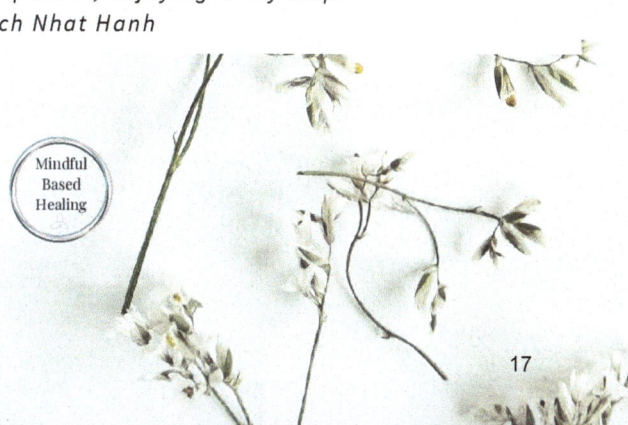

Today's thoughts

Mindful Based Healing

CANCER DEFINED

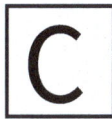 Courage- Often times we don't know how strong or courageous we are until we are challenged.

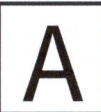 Awareness & Acknowledging- Awareness allows you to process your feelings and proceed with integrity.

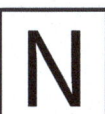 Non-judgement- Think, feel, and do without judging yourself or your feelings. Give yourself grace.

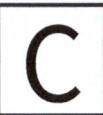 Choose- You have the ability to choose what serves you and let go of what doesn't. Prioritize yourself.

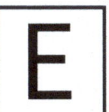 Enjoy- The ability to enjoy life is not defined by the amount of time; rather, how the time is spent.

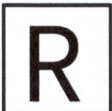 Resiliency- You *are* resilient. You are here, you are brave, you've come this far. You can do it!

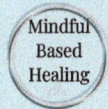

CARE TEAM CONTACTS

....

....

....

....

....

....

SOCIAL SUPPORT CONTACTS

....

....

....

....

....

....

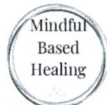

APPOINTMENT   Appointment date:_____

Help your healthcare providers give you the best care possible. Write down questions, take notes, and speak openly about your needs. If you need help or resources to follow the plan....ask!
They can't help you if you don't help yourself.

Concerns	Notes
	_____
	_____
	_____
	_____
	_____

Next steps	What support do I need to succeed?

_____

_____

_____

Follow up

Questions for Care Team

Do I understand my treatment options?

Do I have rides to and from treatment?

Do I have financial support?

Is there support for me to manage my job? Can I cut back?

Is there support for navigating my appointments?

Are there support groups or resources to support me through this diagnosis?

Other:

TREATMENT OPTIONS

DIAGNOSIS: _____

SURGERY

DATE: _____
_____

CHEMO

DATE: _____
_____

RADIATION

DATE: _____

HORMONE THERAPY   **MEDICATIONS**

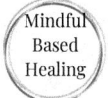

SIDE EFFECTS TO EXPECT

DIAGNOSIS: _____

SURGERY

DATE: _____

CHEMO

DATE: _____

RADIATION

DATE: _____

HORMONE THERAPY

MEDICATIONS

Today's thoughts

Mindful Based Healing

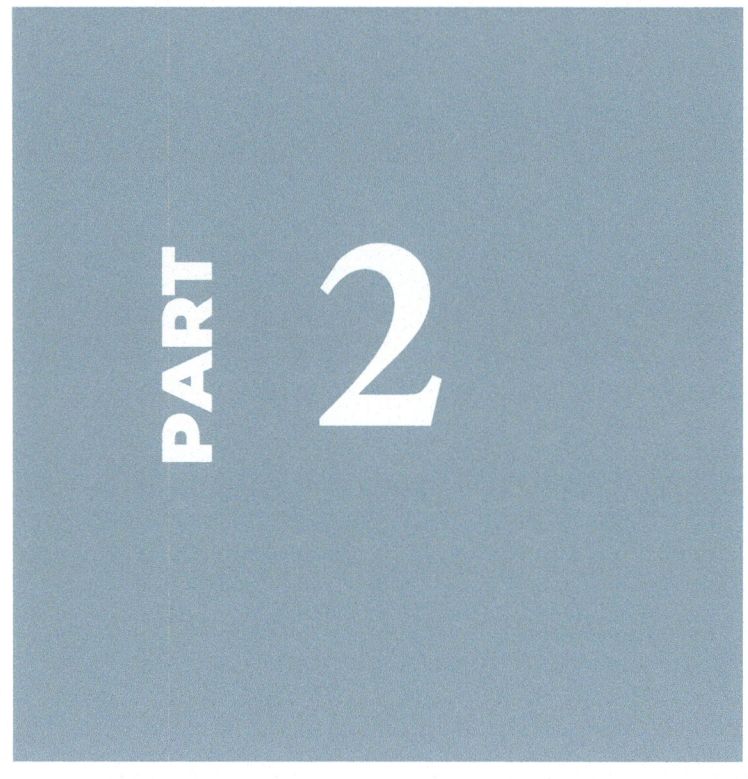

INTRODUCTION TO MINDFULNESS AND BREATHING

Non-judgement

Categorizing things as "good" or "bad" leads to automatic reactions, which can dominate the mind, making it difficult to find peace. Recognize judgement, allow it to unfold and observe your reactions. This allows patterns to be identified without being on autopilot.

INTRODUCTION TO MINDFULNESS

The skills you will learn in this course require you to make changes to mental patterns that may have been with you for some time. Such patterns are usually habitual and automatic, you will only succeed in changing them by putting in time and effort.

A useful attitude is "I'll give this a try with an open mind, at the end of the course I'll decide whether I've learned anything useful and what I can take with me." In order to really know whether this approach can be useful to you, you need to engage with it fully.

An aim of mindfulness is to learn how to be more fully aware and present in each moment. This makes life more enjoyable, interesting, and fulfilling. It means facing up to whatever is present, even when it is unpleasant or difficult, and acknowledging or facing these difficulties. It is, in the long run, the most effective was to reduce unhappiness.

Throughout this guidebook, you will learn gentle and effective tools to cope with difficulties. Be patient and persistent, as you will be working to change deeply established mental patterns. This requires consistency and patience. Nourish yourself. Give it time and you will experience benefits.

In order to receive benefit from these exercises, you don't have to like them; you just have to *do* them.

Today's thoughts

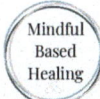

WHAT IS MINDFULNESS?

Mindfulness is the active awareness of this moment in your mind, body, and surroundings, without judgement. Often referred to as *being present*.

Mindfulness is effective in the reduction of stress; which accounts for over 90% of all doctor visits according to the Center for Disease Control (CDC). Stress significantly impacts mental, emotional and physical health, according to the Journal of Health and Social Behavior.

Studies have shown that Mindfulness can have significant health related benefits including:

- better sleep
- stress reduction
- increase levels of T-cell response (improved immune system)
- decrease blood pressure
- decrease risk of heart disease
- decrease emotional reactivity
- reduce cellular aging
- reduce anxiety and depression
- improve coping
- improve pain tolerance
- improve creativity and intuition

*For information regarding sources stated above check out: bit.ly/mindfulhealthcite

EMOTIONS, THOUGHTS OR PHYSICAL SENSATIONS

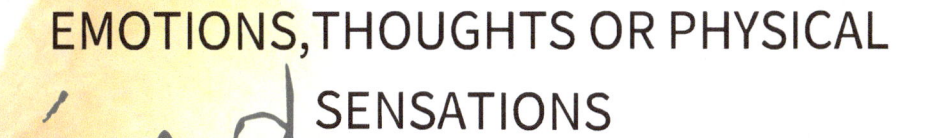

Thoughts that may occur:
- reviewing the past
- planning
- wishing
- comparing
- imagining the future
- analyzing
- labeling
- thinking about others
- circular thinking
- judging the experience

Physical sensations:
- tingly
- burning
- shooting
- prickly
- numb
- shaky
- pounding
- stinging
- pulsing
- throbbing
- dull/sharp
- achy
- trembling
- vibrating
- sinking
- light/heavy
- tense/relaxed
- cool/warm
- clammy/dry
- itchy

Emotions you may experience:
- joy
- surprise
- impatience
- sadness
- fear
- anger
- frustration
- enjoyment
- boredom
- shame
- grief
- pride
- disgust
- anticipation

Today's thoughts

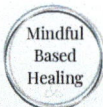

The power of your breath

Practice 1-5 minutes each

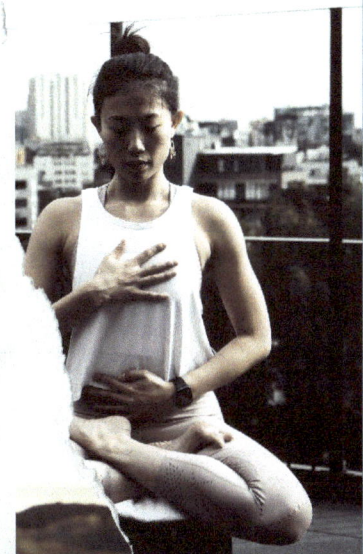

- **Balanced breath** - inhale/ exhale for same length of time (try 4 seconds each)
- **Belly breath** - lying down, place one hand on belly, the other over your heart. Inhale, feel belly rise, exhale pull belly button toward spine
- **2x breath** - exhale is twice as long as inhale (example: inhale 2 seconds/ exhale 4 seconds)
- **Box breath** - inhale/ pause/ exhale/ pause (4 seconds each)
- **Cleansing breath** - inhale through the nose, exhale with open mouth, tongue against back of lower teeth

*Listen to associated audio

> Use breathing techniques as needed. Each technique will support you in a unique way.

Mindful Based Healing

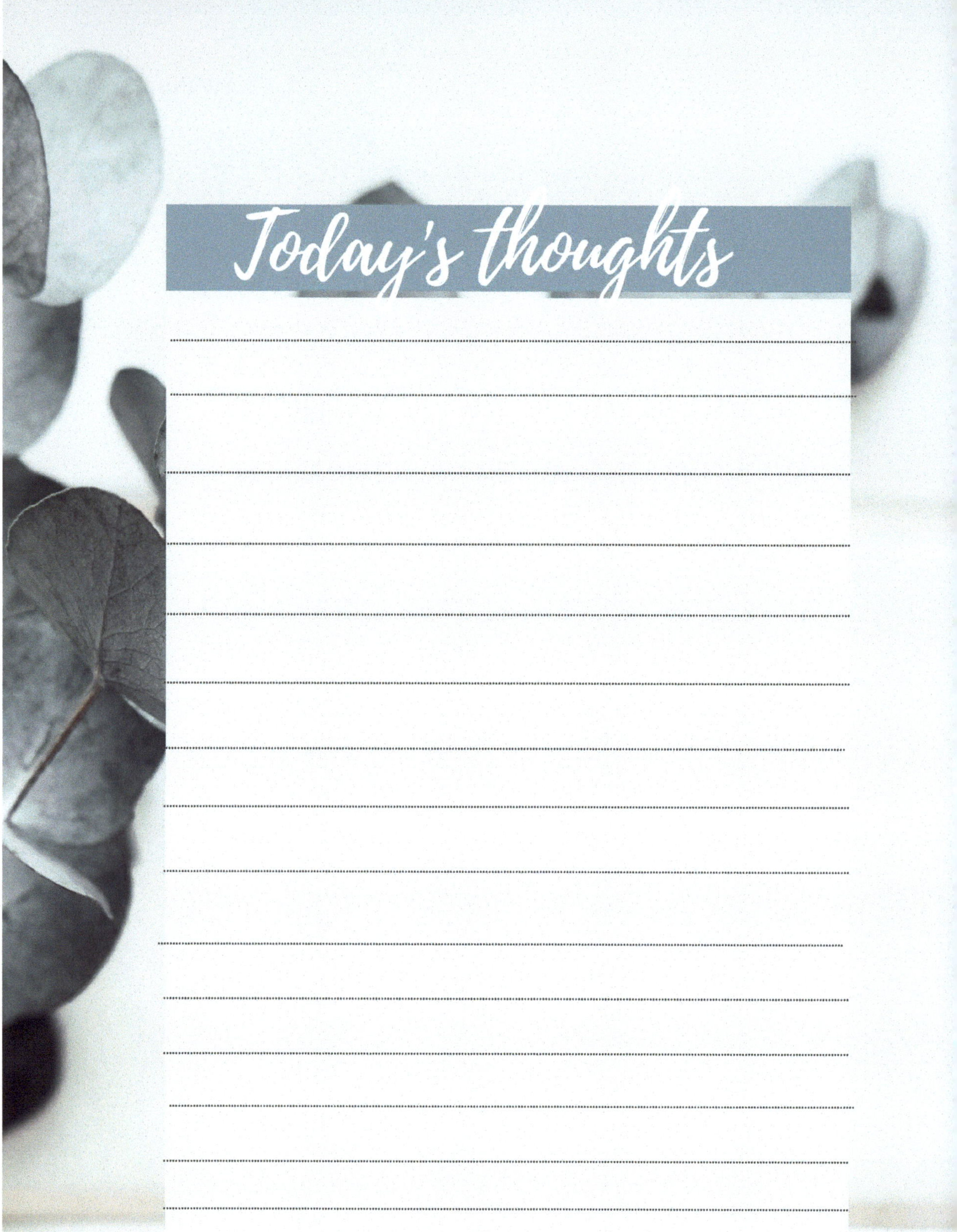

Today's thoughts

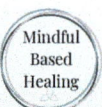

BREATHE OUT PAIN

Inhaling through the nose allows the body to take deeper breaths, which engages the lower lungs. Active lower lungs pump more oxygen into the rest of the body, which results in more support for cells, healthy tissue and organ function.

Practice the breathing exercises on the following page. Play with the speed of inhale/exhale, the depth of the breath as well as the various techniques.

What do you notice? Does one technique serve you in a particular way? As you inhale, notice any areas of discomfort. As you exhale, imagine the pain or discomfort leaving the body with the breath.

Write your experiences below.

WHAT I NOTICE ABOUT BREATH AND PAIN

....
....
....
....
....
....

Today's thoughts

Mindful Based Healing

Body Scan Observations

Sunday :

Monday :

Tuesday :

Wednesday :

Thursday:

Friday :

Saturday :

Mindful Based Healing

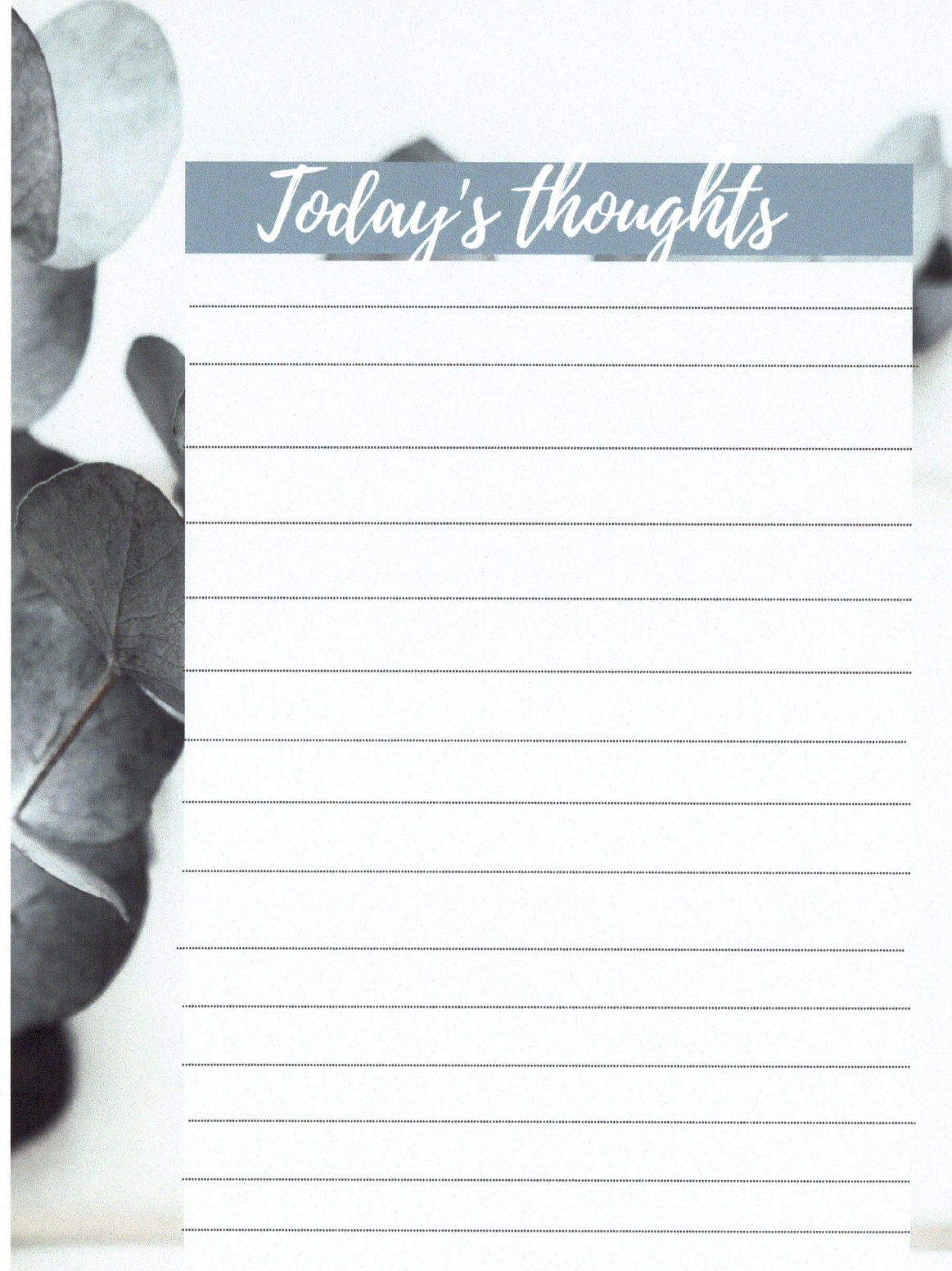

Today's thoughts

Mindful Based Healing

PART 3

MINDFULNESS AND BODY AWARENESS

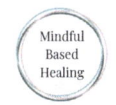

Trust

Develop inner trust. Learn to trust your body and your feelings. Are you pushing past comfort to challenge and grow or are you pushing too hard, leading to overwhelm? Notice discomfort or pain in your body. Notice how it feels to sit with it, but don't allow the sensation to be overpowering. If it doesn't feel good, don't do it. Be safe, choose healthy, live happy.

Today's thoughts

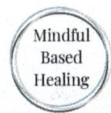

SEVEN DAYS OF MINDFULNESS- PLEASANT EVENTS

In positive psychology research, gratitude is strongly and consistently associated with greater happiness and helps one feel more positive emotions, appreciate good experiences, improve health, deal with adversity, and build strong relationships.

Write down what you are grateful for or perceive as pleasant, including what/where you notice the physical and emotional in the body.

SUNDAY:

MONDAY:

TUESDAY:

WEDNESDAY:

THURSDAY:

FRIDAY:

SATURDAY:

NOTES:

Mindful Based Healing

Today's thoughts

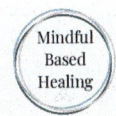

Mindful Based Healing

Don't Wait to be Happy
IF.......
THEN.....

IF _____ happens

THEN _____ (I'll be happy, successful, love myself)

What will you stop waiting for and start enjoying?

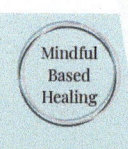

MINDFUL EATING:

Mindful eating is a way to rediscover one of the most pleasurable activities as a human being. It is also a path to uncovering many wonderful activities going on within the body. Mindful eating has the unexpected benefit of helping tap into the body's natural wisdom to really pay attention to how food is supporting or making the body more tired.

Ask questions like:

Am I hungry?
Where do I feel hunger?
What part of me is hungry?
What do I really crave?
What am I tasting just now?
How do I feel after eating a particular food?

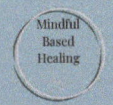

Observations:

Today's thoughts

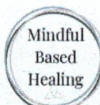

MINDFUL WALKING:

Mindful walking is a way to bring awareness to an activity that is often automatic, without much thought or acknowledgment. It also is a path to uncovering various sensations or emotions going on within the body. Mindful walking can be very therapeutic and beneficial mentally, emotionally and physically.

Ask questions like:
What am I feeling in my body?
Where do I feel support?
What senses are being activated?
What sounds am I hearing?
What is pleasant or unpleasant about this experience?

Observations:

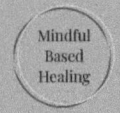

Today's thoughts

THINK BEFORE YOU SPEAK

Your words reflect who you are. They have the power to influence how you are perceived as well as the merit to what you are saying. Words are used to either help or hurt yourself and others. Choose them carefully.

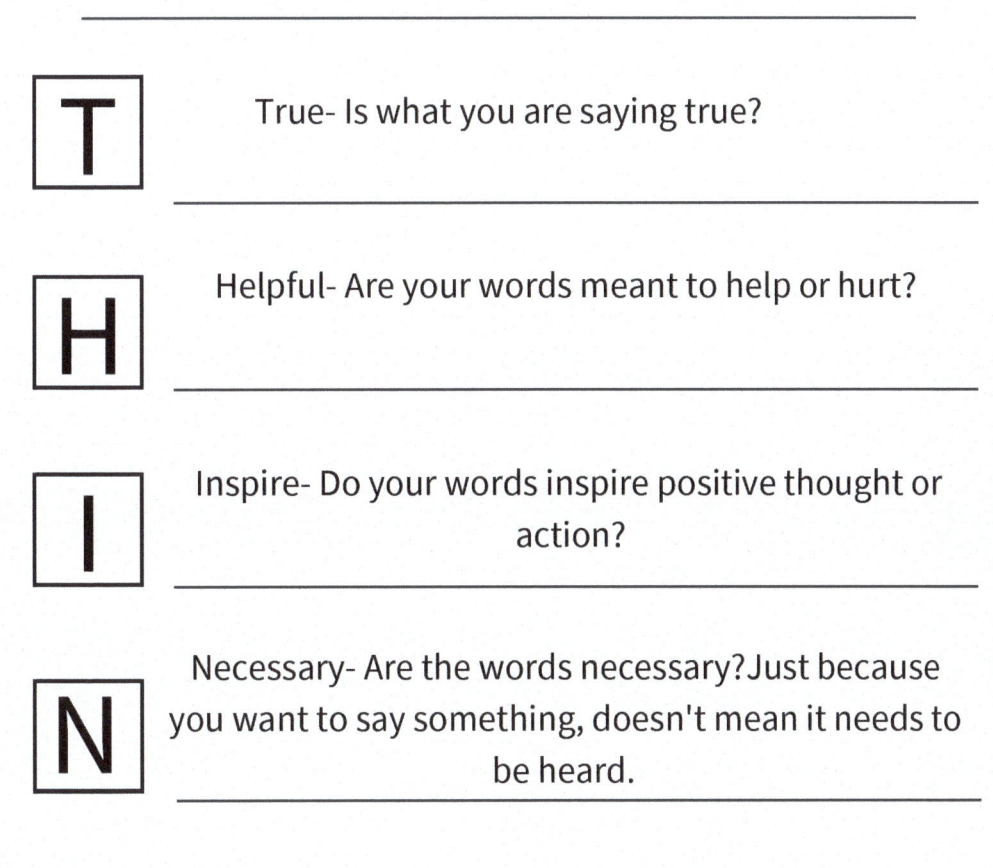

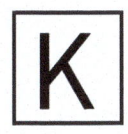

T — True- Is what you are saying true?

H — Helpful- Are your words meant to help or hurt?

I — Inspire- Do your words inspire positive thought or action?

N — Necessary- Are the words necessary? Just because you want to say something, doesn't mean it needs to be heard.

K — Kind- Are your words kind? If not, what is the purpose behind them?

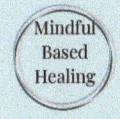

Mindful Based Healing

Today's thoughts

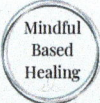

MINDFUL BODY TRACKER

As you begin to be more present, you may be more aware of how food, medication or activity affects your body. Take note on how you are fueling and supporting your body during this time.

When I (eat/ drink/ move/ take):	My body feels:

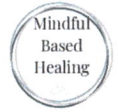

Today's thoughts

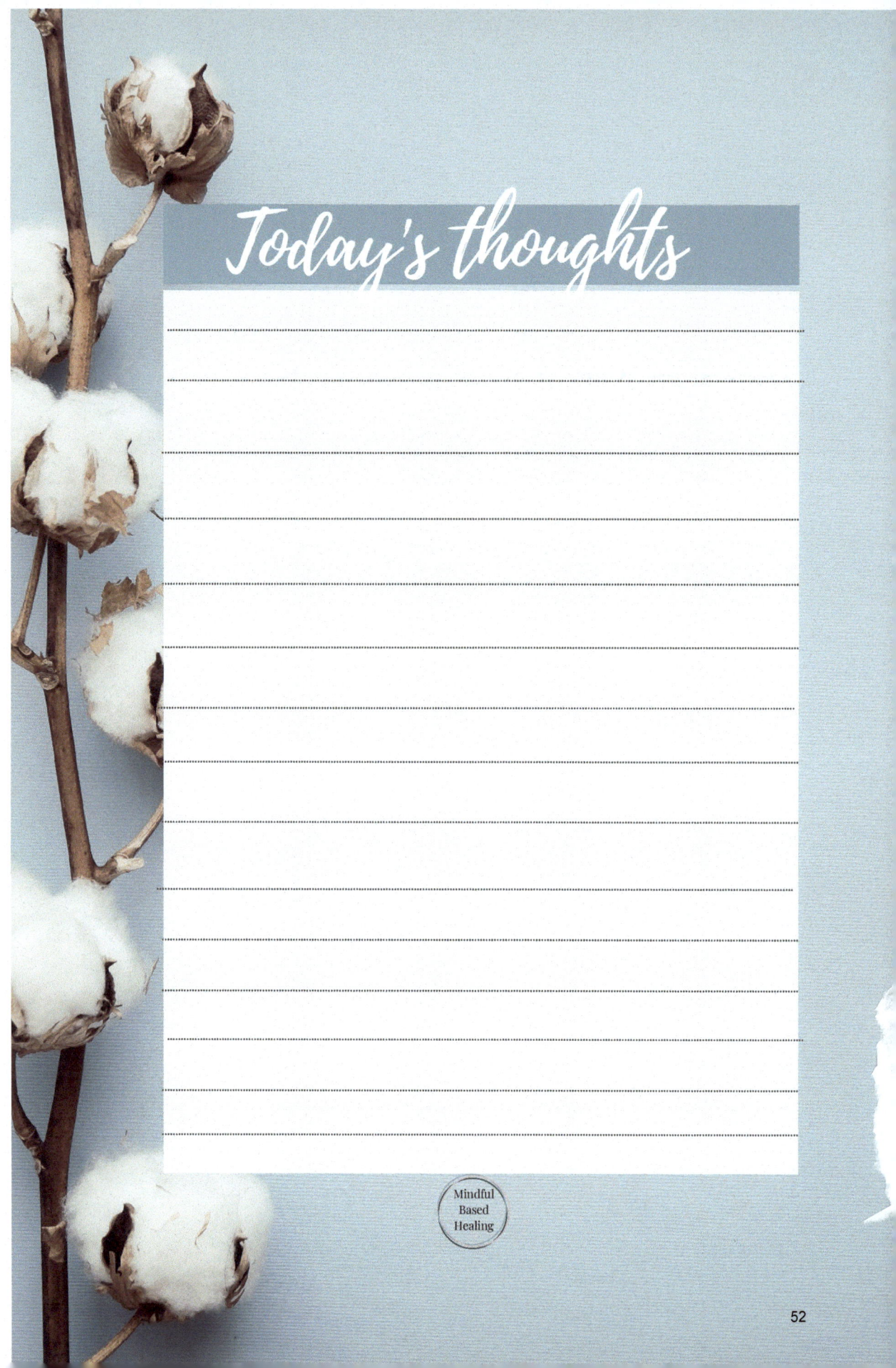

Mindful Based Healing

EMOTIONS COLOR LIFE

Emotions can impact how a situation or information is perceived.
Track your feelings throughout the month(s) through color (add your own emotions)

PINK	RED	ORANGE	YELLOW	GREEN	BLUE	PURPLE
Creative Energetic	Angry Irritable	Pain Stressed	Positive Happy	Sick Exhausted	Sad Depressed	Calm Content

Mindful Based Healing

Today's thoughts

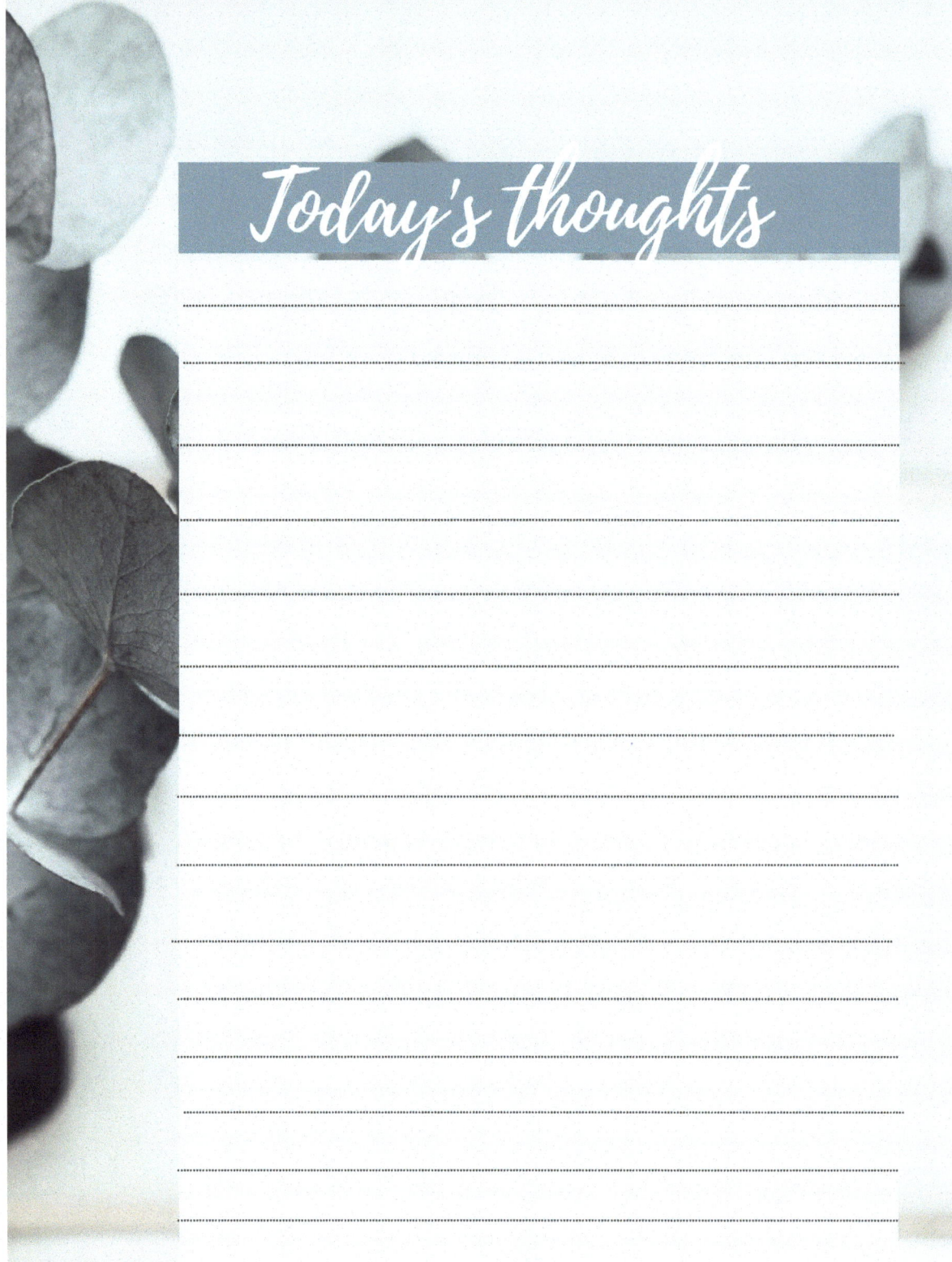

HOW I *THINK*

How I used my words to make a difference.

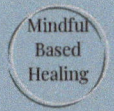

| T |
| H |
| I |
| N |
| K |

PART 4

TYPES OF STRESS AND EFFECT ON HEALTH

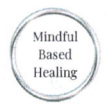

Letting go

Holding on too tightly to what you wish for can prevent growth and acceptance. For example, in preparation for upcoming test results or doctor appointment, you most likely want the results to show your cancer is gone, that you're in remission. Whether you worry, stress and think about this over and over, the test results will show what they show. Worrying about them will not change the outcome but it can negatively affect your health, well-being, and quality of life in the meantime. Try to focus on what is, what you are capable of, and how you can enjoy life while you are waiting for results.

Today's thoughts

SEVEN DAYS OF MINDFULNESS- UNPLEASANT EVENTS

Bringing awareness to what is perceived as an unpleasant situation or experience is important in identifying patterns, behaviors and coping mechanisms. Paying attention to *why* it is perceived as unpleasant allows one to choose how to proceed.

Write down what you perceive as unpleasant, including what/where you notice the physical and emotional in the body.

SUNDAY:

MONDAY:

TUESDAY:

WEDNESDAY:

THURSDAY:

FRIDAY:

SATURDAY:

NOTES:

Mindful Based Healing

Today's thoughts

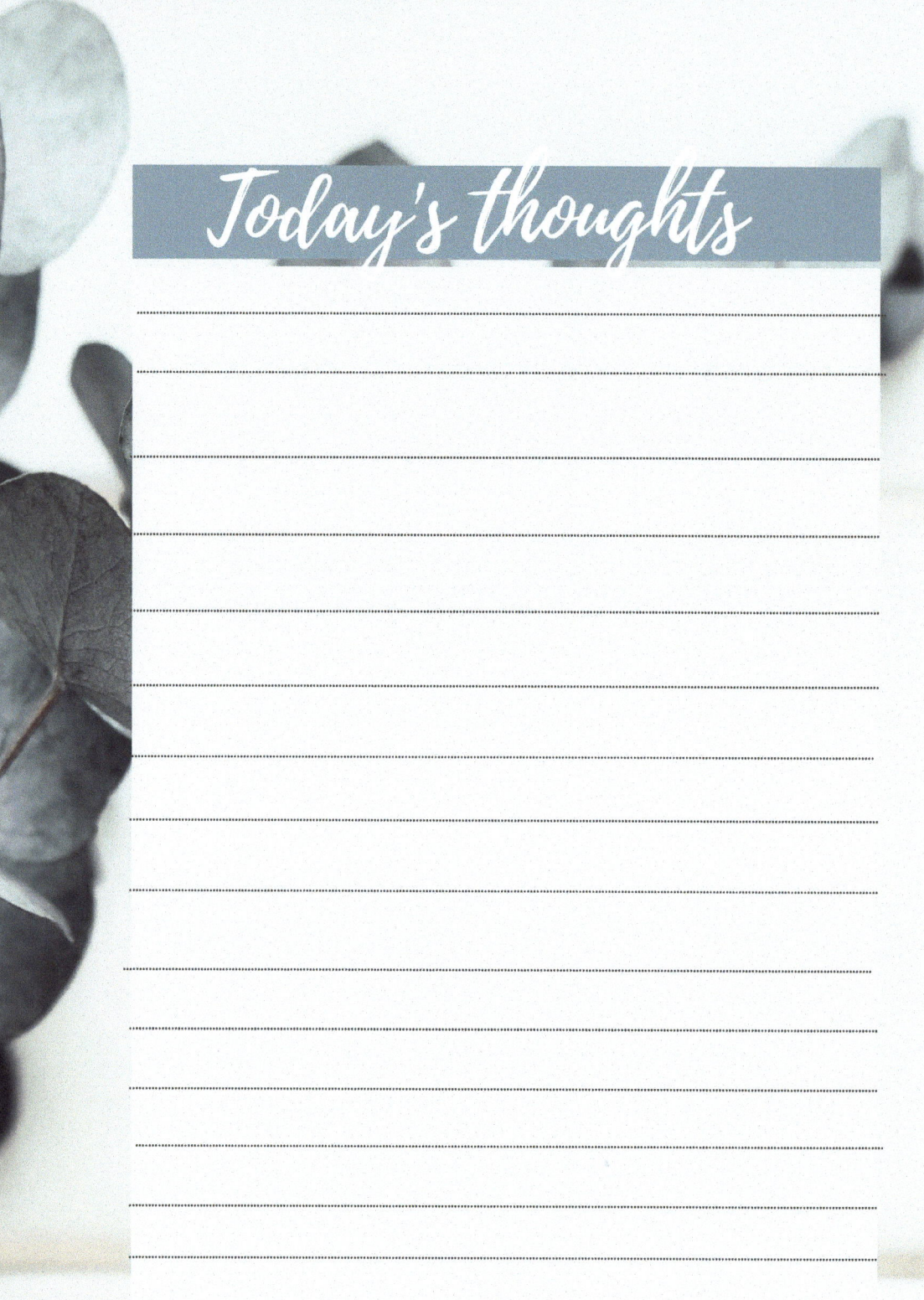

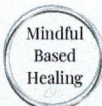

STRESS AND EFFECTS ON HEALTH

TYPES OF STRESS

- **Physical stress:** trauma such as high blood pressure, changes in weight, frequent colds or infections, and changes in the menstrual cycle and libido

- **Mental or cognitive stress:** difficulty concentrating,e worrying, anxiety, and trouble remembering, a sense of loss of control.
-
    Emotional stress: being angry, irritated, moody, or frustrated,
    crisis of values, meaning, and purpose; a misalignment with one's core beliefs.

EFFECTS OF STRESS

- Increased duration and release of hormones like adrenaline and cortisol
- Increased heart rate
- Slower digestion
- Restricted blood flow to major muscle groups
- Changes various other autonomic nervous functions
- Increased risk of anxiety and depression
- Sleep disturbance
- High blood pressure
- Headaches
- Heart disease

COMMON SYSTEMS EFFECTED BY STRESS

- musculoskeletal
- respiratory
- cardiovascular
- endocrine

- gastrointestinal
- nervous
- reproductive

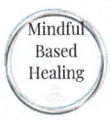

Today's thoughts

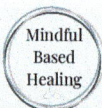

Mindful Based Healing

STRESS AND EFFECTS ON HEALTH

TYPES OF STRESS

- **Physical stress:** trauma such as high blood pressure, changes in weight, frequent colds or infections, and changes in the menstrual cycle and libido

- **Mental or cognitive stress:** difficulty concentrating,e worrying, anxiety, and trouble remembering, a sense of loss of control.
-
  Emotional stress: being angry, irritated, moody, or frustrated,
  crisis of values, meaning, and purpose; a misalignment with one's core beliefs.

EFFECTS OF STRESS

- Increased duration and release of hormones like adrenaline and cortisol
- Increased heart rate
- Slower digestion
- Restricted blood flow to major muscle groups
- Changes various other autonomic nervous functions
- Increased risk of anxiety and depression
- Sleep disturbance
- High blood pressure
- Headaches
- Heart disease

COMMON SYSTEMS EFFECTED BY STRESS

- musculoskeletal
- respiratory
- cardiovascular
- endocrine

- gastrointestinal
- nervous
- reproductive

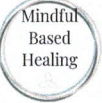

61

Today's thoughts

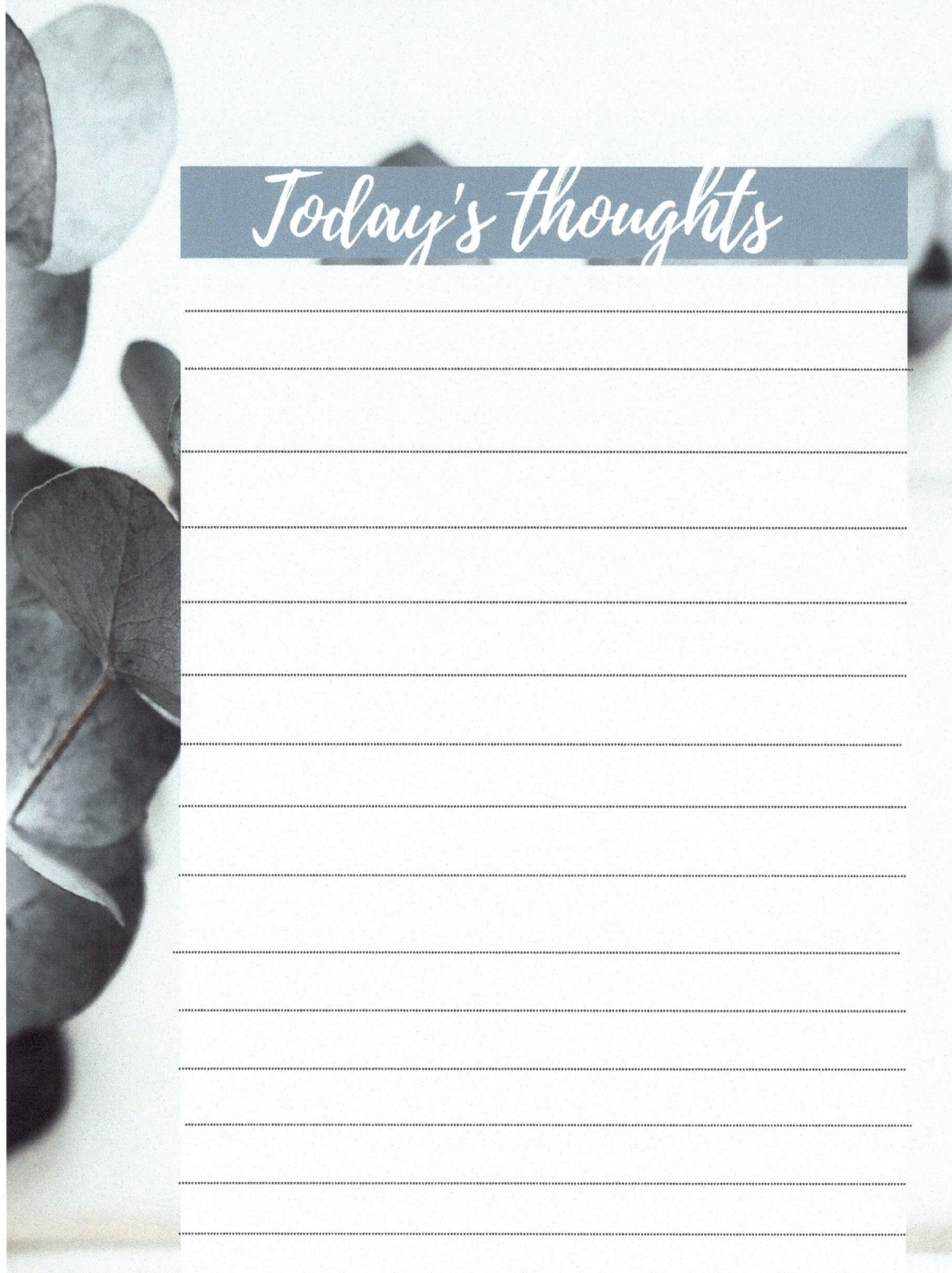

COMFORT, GROWTH OR OVERWHELM?

Beyond the comfort zone is a space for growth, to push beyond what is comfortable to a space that challenges one to be better. Beyond growth can be a place of overwhelm if there is lack of awareness or self-care. Notice the thoughts, emotions and physical sensations occurring in the body throughout your healing journey.

Lack of self-care = Overwhelm zone

Challenge = Growth zone

Comfort zone

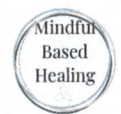

Mindful Based Healing

Today's thoughts

Mindful Based Healing

RESPONDING TO EMOTIONAL OR PHYSICAL PAIN
Blocking / Drowning / Letting Go / Turning Toward
inspired by Dave Potter

The two most typical responses to significant pain, whether primarily physical or emotional, are **Blocking** and **Drowning**. In "Blocking", one pushes away or denies discomfort by numbing, distracting or staying busy, convincing oneself there isn't a problem, or by self-medicating with food, alcohol, or drugs. This "solution" is problematic, not just because of unwanted side-effects, but because nothing has been done to resolve the underlying cause of the pain.

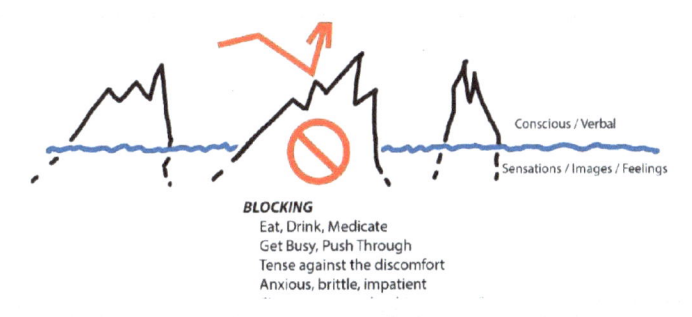

BLOCKING
Eat, Drink, Medicate
Get Busy, Push Through
Tense against the discomfort
Anxious, brittle, impatient

The second typical response, "Drowning", is not a conscious choice, but the effect of not having sufficient resources to deal with the painful condition. In Drowning, one is consumed by the difficulty, overwhelmed with the discomfort and its associated fears or judgments. Accompanying the physical or emotional pain often come feelings of helplessness and judgment ("I can't do this!", "What if this gets worse?", "How could they/I have been so stupid?!?", etc.). In the end, one feels hopeless and powerless about how to take care of the pain.

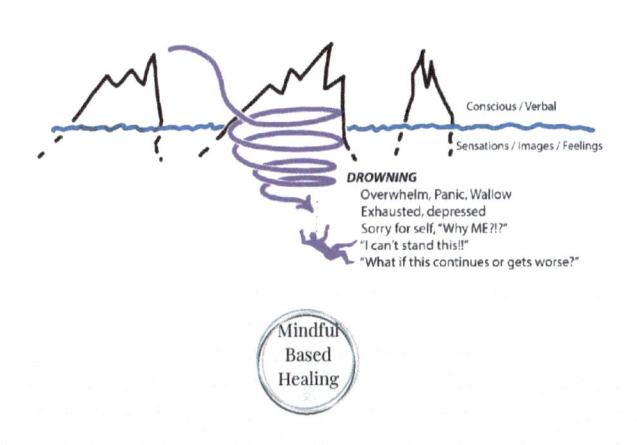

DROWNING
Overwhelm, Panic, Wallow
Exhausted, depressed
Sorry for self, "Why ME?!?"
"I can't stand this!!"
"What if this continues or gets worse?"

Mindful Based Healing

RESPONDING TO EMOTIONAL OR PHYSICAL PAIN
Blocking / Drowning / Letting Go / Turning Toward continued

There is another approach, called "Turning Toward". This is a powerful method, but it is deeply counter-intuitive, because the last thing one may want to do; move closer to the perceived trouble. Instead of moving away from the difficulty, move toward it. Although such an exploration might sound scary and uncomfortable, this can be a gentle process that draws on the skills of awareness and non-judgment which have been strengthening throughout this course.

In "Turning Toward", there is an attitude of open curiosity and a willingness to be with and explore what is being encountered, even if it is uncomfortable and the discomfort may lessen, or even disappears.

TURNING TOWARD
Attitude of Open Curiosity
Willingness to be with "What Is"
Befriending and Exploring

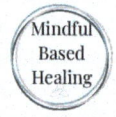

Mindful Based Healing

RESPONDING TO EMOTIONAL OR PHYSICAL PAIN
Blocking / Drowning / Letting Go / Turning Toward continued

Often, it's not just blocking or drowning, but a swinging from one to the other. For instance, after a period of overwhelm *(drowning)*, there can be a retreat into eating or self-medicating *(blocking)*, which is only effective temporarily, then another round of overwhelming emotion begins *(drowning)*, and when that is too much, there's escape with distraction *(blocking)*, and so on. This can be a never- ending cycle.

When some difficulty presents itself during meditation in the form of a thought, emotion, or physical sensation, simply acknowledge it and then "gently" return to the object of awareness (breath or mantra). This is called "Letting Go and Returning":

This approach strengthens grounding, stability and resilience, and can lead to pleasant, even blissful states. If the acknowledgment is done in a truly non-reactive way, the difficulty may actually shift or dissolve. This may take practice and one may notice strong emotions or de-stressing taking place over a period of days or weeks. Get support and be consistent, the de-stressing and strong emotions will pass as they leave the body.

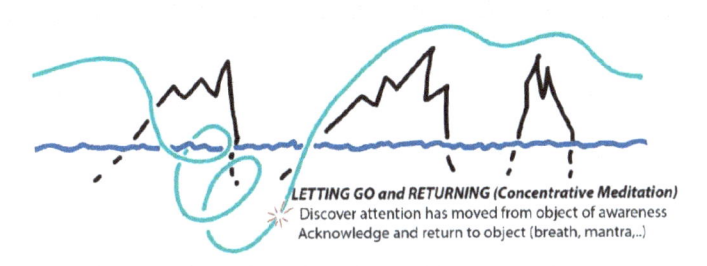

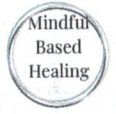

LETTING GO and RETURNING (Concentrative Meditation)
Discover attention has moved from object of awareness
Acknowledge and return to object (breath, mantra,...)

Mindful Based Healing

Today's thoughts

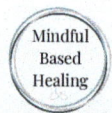

PART 5

PATTERNS, BARRIERS AND COPING

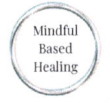

Practice Patience

Practice patience in every situation. The experiences are happening anyway, so allow yourself to be patient, allow the situation to unfold in its own time, and experience clarity and calm rather than helplessness or anger.

Today's thoughts

3 P's

Use 3P's or STOP to bring awareness to the present moment. Begin with 1-10 minutes and use as many times as needed daily.

----

1. PAUSE
Stop,
take a breath,
notice the moment,
without reacting

3. PROCEED
Choose words and actions that support your values and serve you in this moment.

2. Be PRESENT
Bring body awareness to physical sensations, thoughts and emotions

Practice
How did the 3P's support me today?

Observations

Mindful Based Healing

Today's thoughts

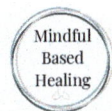

Mindful Based Healing

IDENTIFY STRESS COPING PATTERNS
(above the line: common, traditional, non-creative - one or both parties get less than they want)

① DEMAND: Hold firm (fight)
What I need/want is most important
"My way or the highway"
Express as: anger, rage, fury, upset, annoyed, frustration, irritable, oppositional, argumentative, bullying, aggressive
Leads to emotional intensity
I satisfy my needs at the expense of yours.

② ACCOMMODATE: Passive (freeze)
What you need/want is most important
"Don't make waves"
Give in, conform to reduce conflict
Express as: grief, loss, shame, sad, depressed, helpless, hopeless, numb, disconnected, withdrawn, poor eye contact
Leads to emotional blunting
I satisfy your needs at the expense of my own.

③ WITHDRAW: Walk Away/ retreat (flight)
It's too difficult to deal with
"I don't care"
Withdraw, avoid, retreat, ignore, deny, or suppress
Express as: panic, fear, anxiety, dread, worry, excuse-making, avoiding, changing the subject, deflecting/distracting, easily startled
Leads to emotional liability
Neither you nor I satisfy our needs.

④ COMPROMISE: Tend/ befriend (fixing)
Moderately demanding/ accommodating
"I give some, you give some"; "split the difference"
Express as: rescuing, enabling, co-dependency, unhealthy attachment, over-extending, people-pleasing, caregiver-burnout
Leads to emotional exhaustion
We each give up some needs to satisfy the other.

(below the line: rare, more difficult, but much more powerful - root goals of both parties satisfied)

⑤ BLEND: Both get needs met
Requires mindful awareness and exploration of:
Behavior (body language, tone) / Feelings / Needs (both yours and theirs)
Three steps are involved:
1. Recognition and acceptance of both party's feelings and perceived needs
2. Discovery and inquiry into other party's intentions and goals
3. Mutual exploration of potential solutions satisfying intention and goals of both parties

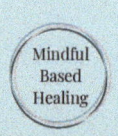

Mindful Based Healing

IDENTIFY PATTERNS

In order to make changes, one must first recognize patterns of behavior. Once patterns are identified, you then have the power to choose which patterns serve you and which you choose to change.

WHEN I AM UPSET, I:

WHEN I AM EXCITED, I:

WHEN I AM AFRAID, I:

WHEN I AM HAPPY, I:

WHEN I FEEL ALONE, I:

WHEN I FEEL SUPPORTED, I:

Today's thoughts

Mindful Based Healing

STOP

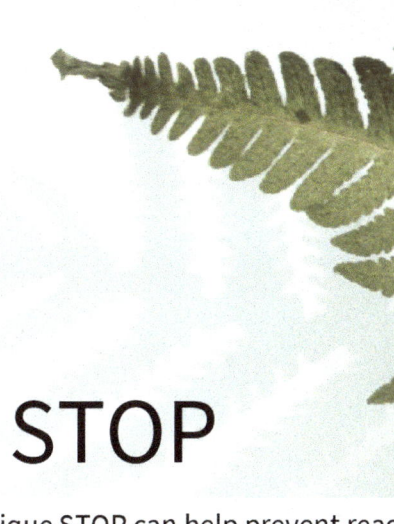

The Mindfulness technique STOP can help prevent reaction by acknowledging and slowing down, allowing space to reconnect with mind, body, and heart. This provides for a more thoughtful and intuitive response. Write down what thoughts, emotions of physical response you notice.

Technique	Experience
S- Stop what you're doing, notice how you feel	
T- Take a breath, bring attention to breath for one minute	
O- Observe, expanding awareness outward: sights, sounds, smells	
P- Proceed in a way true to your values with new possibilities and without expectation	

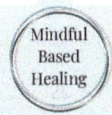

Mindful Based Healing

BARRIERS TO SUCCESS

Your care team has goals for you including nutrition, medications, treaments, etc. What is preventing you from following the plan? What support do you need in order to succeed? Identify your barriers and discuss with your Care Team to ensure success in your care plan.

Barrier 1

Actions I can take:

Barrier 2

Actions I can take:

Barrier 3

Actions I can take:

Barrier 4

Actions I can take:

Mindful Based Healing

Today's thoughts

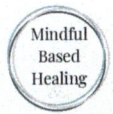

Mindful Based Healing

COPING WITH STRESS

Work, financials, upcoming appointments or tests can cause physical and emotional distress. Instead of focusing on the stressor and allowing it to control you; acknowledge it, feel your feelings, and focus on what you can control.

I AM STRESSED ABOUT:

I WILL FOCUS ON:

I AM ANXIOUS ABOUT:

I WILL SUPPORT MYSELF BY:

I FEEL:

I WILL:

Mindful Based Healing

Today's thoughts

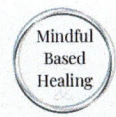

RAIN

R—Recognize What's Going On
Recognize means consciously acknowledging thoughts, feelings, or behaviors that are affecting you. This can be a done with a simple mental whisper, noting what you are most aware of.

A—Allow the Experience to be There, as is, without trying to fix or avoid it.
Allowing the thoughts, emotions, feelings, or sensations you have recognized, pause to deepen attention and perhaps whisper "it's ok", "this belongs", or "yes."

I—Investigate with Interest and Care
To investigate, call on natural curiosity with the desire to know truth, and direct a more focused attention to the present experience.
Perhaps ask yourself: *What most wants attention? How am I experiencing this in my body? What am I believing? What does this want from me? What does it most need?*
Whatever the inquiry, your investigation will be most transformational if you shift from conceptualizing to bringing awareness to the *feelings* in the body.

N—Nurture with Self-Compassion
Self-compassion may naturally arise when you recognize you are suffering.
Try to sense what the wounded, frightened or hurting place inside needs most, then practice self-care or loving-kindness. *Does it need a message of reassurance? Of forgiveness? Of companionship? Of love?*
Experiment which gesture of self-care or loving-kindness offers comfort, support or awareness. It may be the mental whisper, "I'm here". "I'm sorry". "I love you". "I'm listening". "It's not my fault".
Many people find comfort or healing by gently placing a hand on the heart; or by envisioning being embraced by warm, radiant light. If it feels difficult to offer yourself love, imagine a loving figure, family member, friend or pet offering love to you.

After the RAIN
After completing the active steps of RAIN, it's important to notice the quality of your own presence and rest in the space of awareness.
The benefit of RAIN is realizing that you are no longer imprisoned by or identified with any limiting sense of self. Give yourself the gift of awareness and freedom that come from listening to your inner truth.

PART 6

POWER OF POSITIVE THINKING

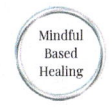

THE POWER OF A HUG

EVERYONE NEEDS A HUG

There were twin brothers tragically separated at birth. One given to a loving family, the other with two parents, food and a bed, but there was emptiness inside him. The boy in the loving home grew to be happy and well-adjusted, while the other became angry and quick to argue. He heard more than once,
"we don't hug in this family."

THE GIFT OF CANCER

"One of the gifts of cancer is the breaking down of barriers throughout my life. One example, I now have more opportunities to share a hug throughout the week. Cancer has given me many opportunities to give and receive; to share a hug. I've come to learn one does not have to be a family member or close friend. Heck, there are occasions when the time is right to give someone a hug and I don't even know his or her name. A hug is simple, yet powerful and healing." - Ron (former patient)

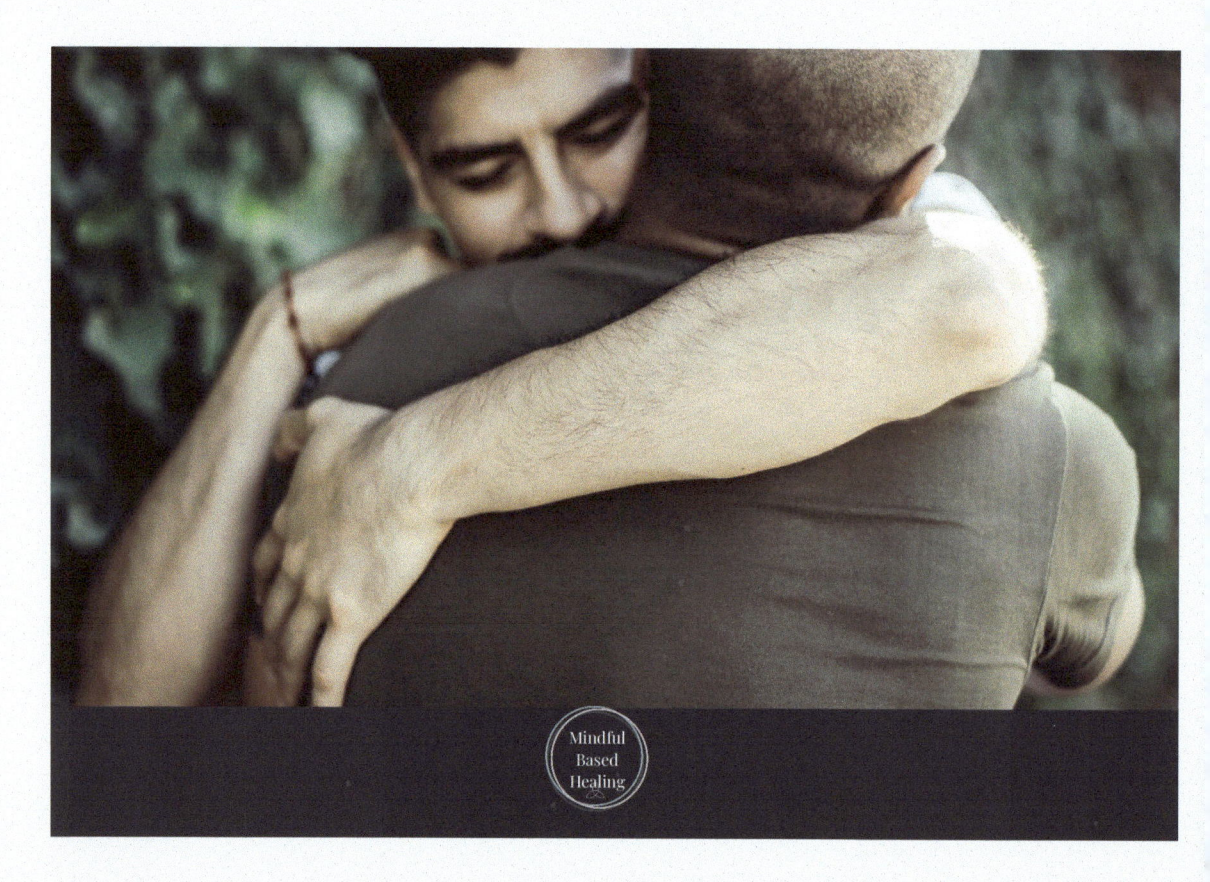

Today's thoughts

Mindful Based Healing

Mindset matters

"If you think you can, you are right. If you think you can't, you are right."

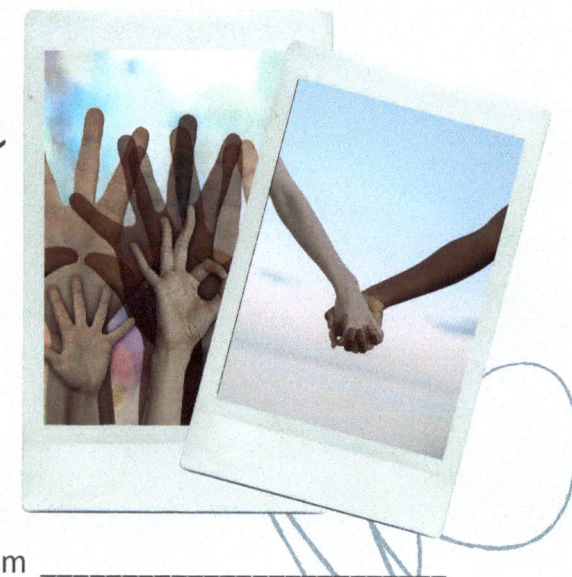

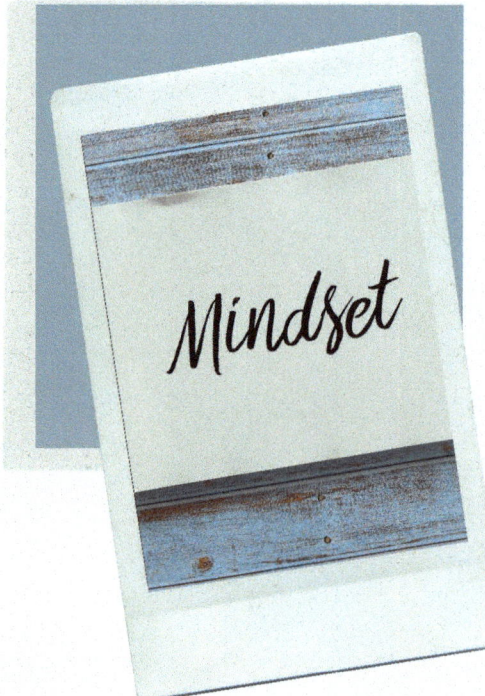

When I am _____
I feel it physically in my _____
I notice my body reacts by
_____.
I use _____ to bring back my awareness and use
_____ as my anchor.
Patterns I am noticing include
_____.
Are they serving me?
_____
Alternative techniques I can try include
_____

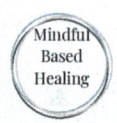

Mindful Based Healing

SELF-CARE TRACKER

Track your self-care activites with color throughout your journey. The more present you become, the more you may notice you choose to prioritize your well-being.

	Sunday(s)	Monday(s)	Tuesday(s)	Wednesday(s)	Thursday(s)	Friday(s)	Saturday(s)
Mindful movement							
Healthy meals							
Drink water							
Smile or laugh daily							
Practice gratitude							
Mindful breathing							
Getting enough rest							

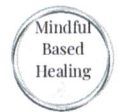

Mindful Based Healing

Today's thoughts

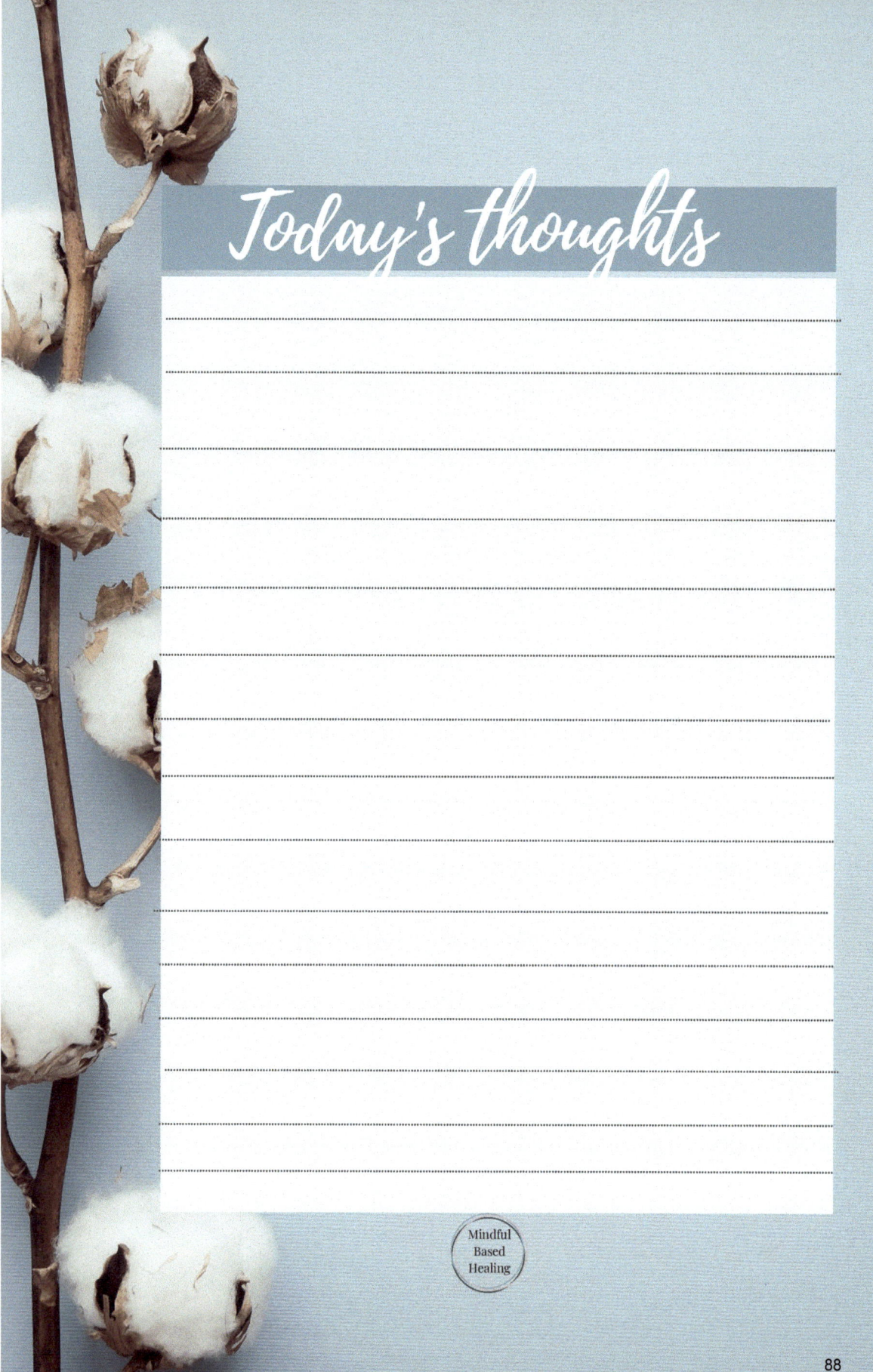

Mindful Based Healing

POWER OF POSITIVE THOUGHTS

There is power in positivity. Rather than moving away *from* uncomfortable, negative, or unpleasant; try moving *toward* the positive, pleasant, and comfortable. This shift in mindset trains your brain to begin finding the positive in situations or feelings. This shift can help you de-stress and make room for a more enjoyable life.

Instead of: Moving *from* unpleasant thoughts *"I don't want to talk to this person"*	Try: Shift *toward* more pleasant thoughts *"I'm going to join that conversation"*

Mindful Based Healing

Today's thoughts

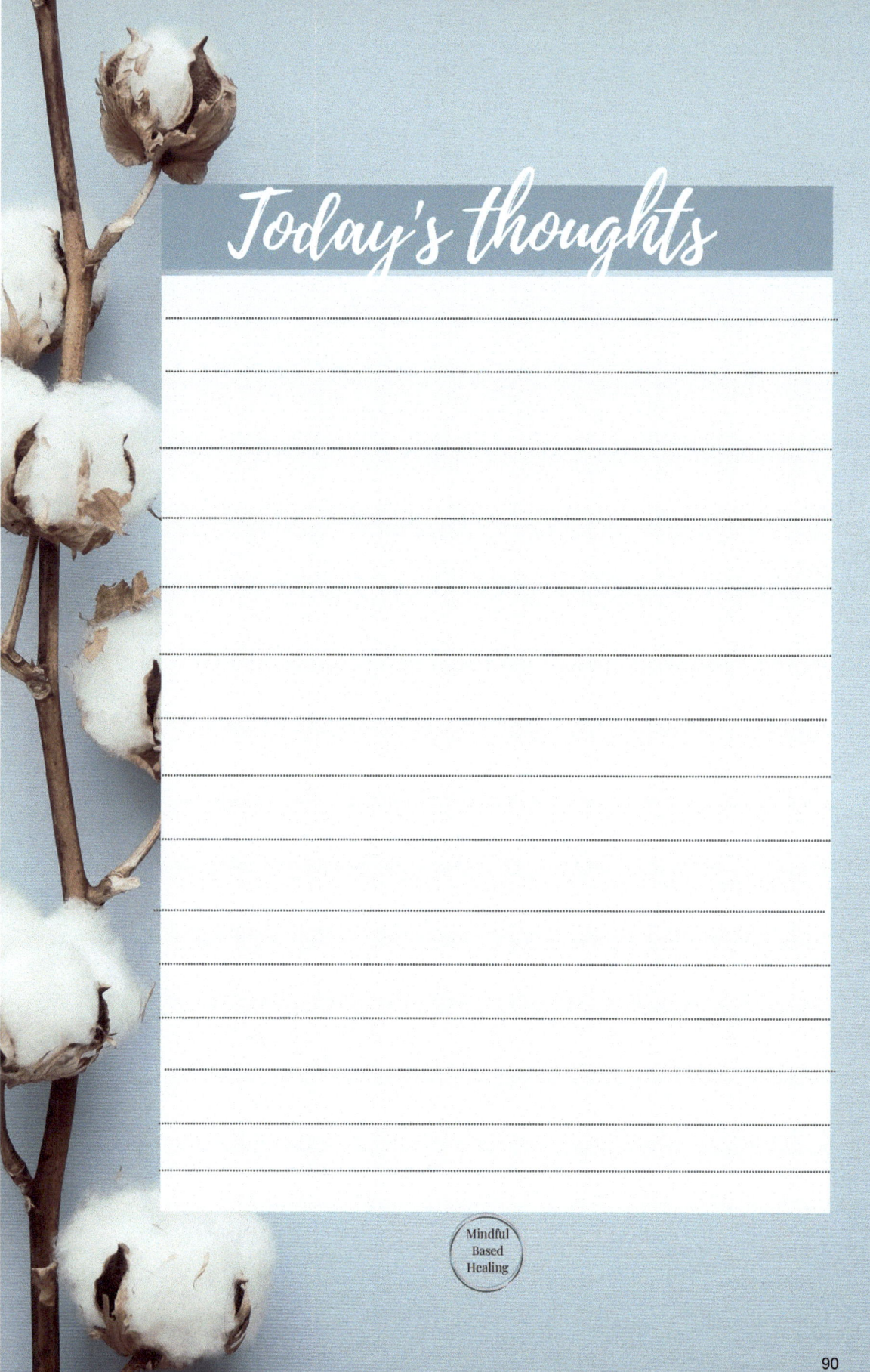

LOVE AFTER LOVE

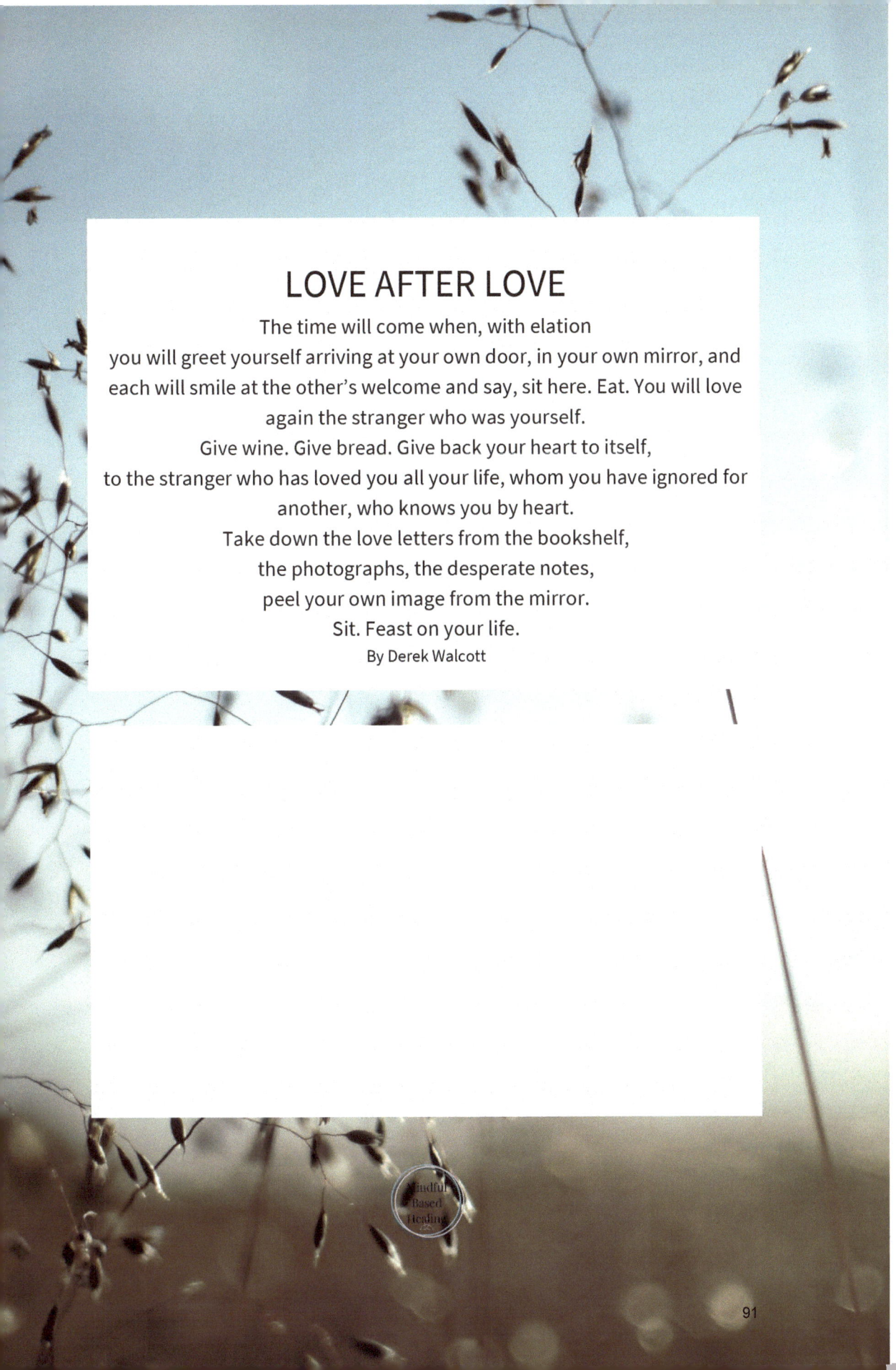

The time will come when, with elation
you will greet yourself arriving at your own door, in your own mirror, and
each will smile at the other's welcome and say, sit here. Eat. You will love
again the stranger who was yourself.
Give wine. Give bread. Give back your heart to itself,
to the stranger who has loved you all your life, whom you have ignored for
another, who knows you by heart.
Take down the love letters from the bookshelf,
the photographs, the desperate notes,
peel your own image from the mirror.
Sit. Feast on your life.
By Derek Walcott

Today's thoughts

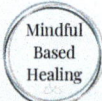

The gift of letting go

Better to be good than perfect,
Better to be done than good,
Better to try than be done.
Don't let perfection stop you from enjoying your life.

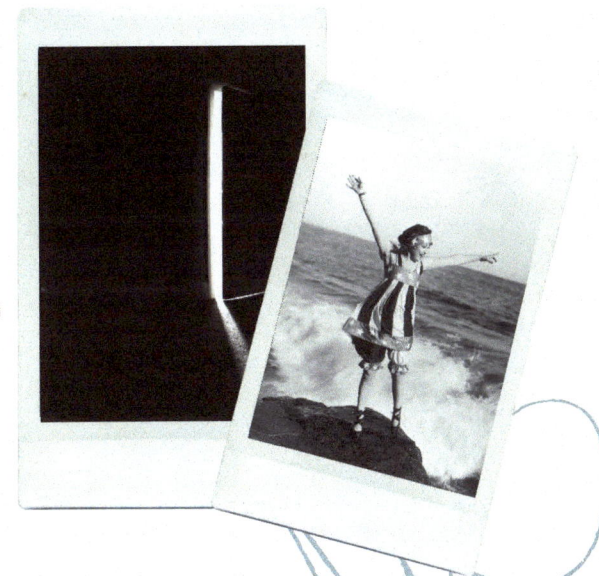

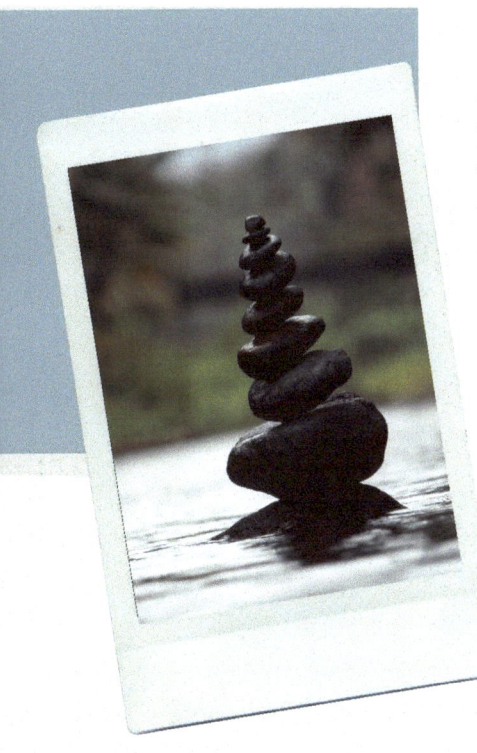

"The longer I live, the more I realize the impact of attitude on life. Attitude to me is more important than facts. It is more important than the past, than education, than money, than circumstances, than failures, than successes, than what other people think or say or do. It is more important than appearance, giftedness or skill. It will make or break a company…a church… a home. The remarkable thing is you have a choice every day regarding the attitude you will embrace for that day. We cannot change our past. We cannot change the fact that people will act in a certain way. We cannot change the inevitable. The only thing we can do is play on the one string we have, and that is our attitude. I am convinced that life is 10% what happens to me and 90% how I respond to it". ~ Charles Swindoll

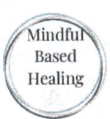

Mindful Based Healing

Today's thoughts

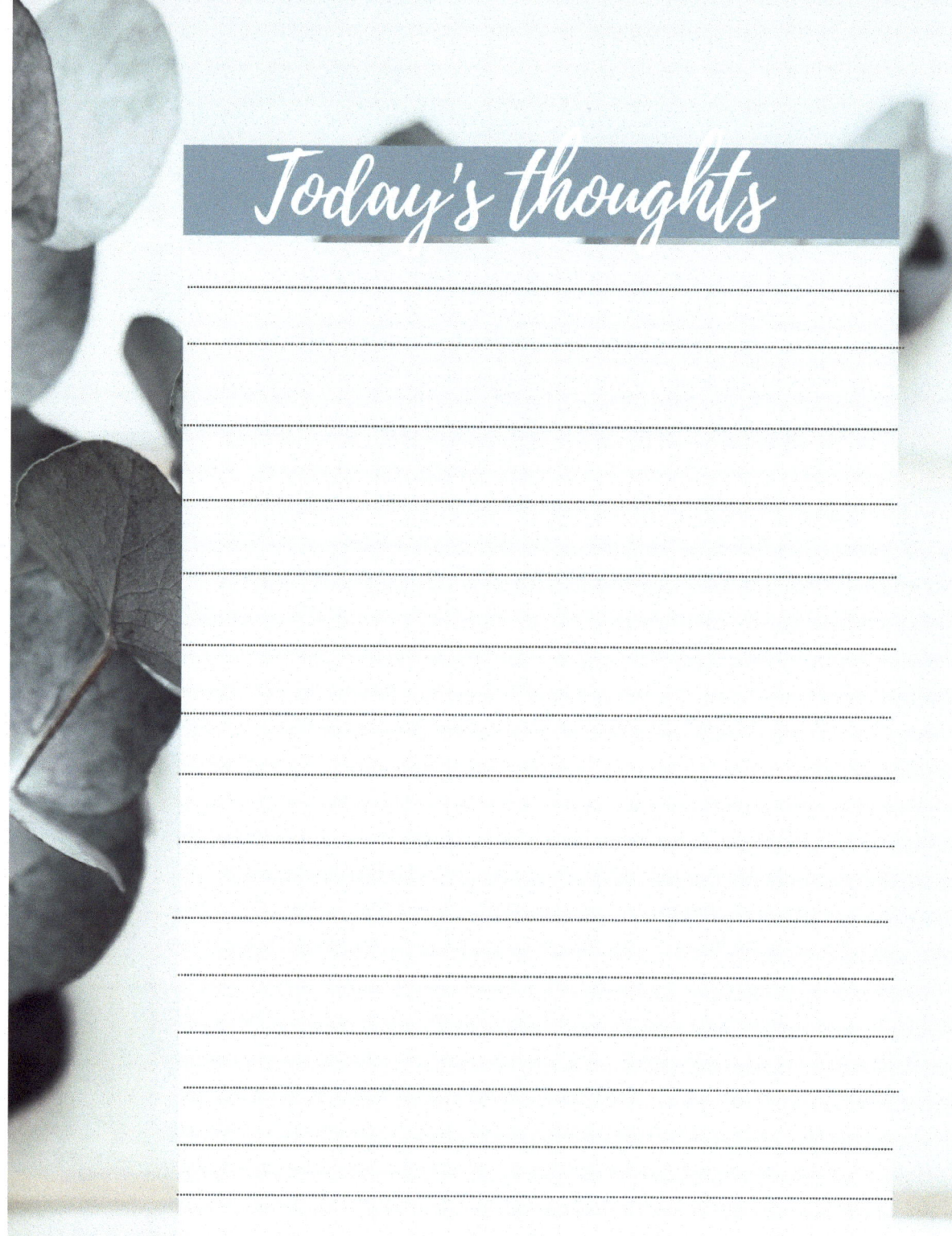

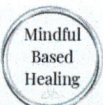

LOVING KINDNESS SCRIPT
continued

Sending Loving-Kindness to All Living Beings

Now expand your awareness and picture the whole globe in front of you as a little ball.

Send warm wishes to all living beings, who, like you, want to be happy:

May you be happy, may you be healthy, may you live with ease.
May you be happy, may you be healthy, may you live with ease.
May you be happy, may you be healthy, may you live with ease.

Sending Loving-Kindness to Yourself

Now bring your awareness inward. Notice your state of mind, your physical body. Do you feel lighter, happier?

Send warm wishes and love to yourself:
I love you, I appreciate you, I forgive you.
May I be happy, may I be healthy, may I live with ease.
I love you, I appreciate you, I forgive you.
May I be happy, may I be healthy, may I live with ease.
I love you, I appreciate you, I forgive you.
May I be happy, may I be healthy, may I live with ease.

Repeat as needed to send forgiveness, kindness, and love.

Take a deep breath in. And breathe out. And another deep breath in and let it go. Notice the state of your mind and how you feel.

When you're ready, allow your eyes to open.

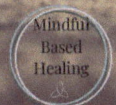

LOVING KINDNESS SCRIPT
continued

Sending Loving-Kindness to Loved Ones

Now imagine someone you care deeply about. Picture him/her standing in front of you whether they are in your life currently or from the past. Imagine you can touch, embrace and send love to that person. Feel love flow from you to this person through your emabrace, through your thoughts and through your words.

Repeat the following phrases, silently:
May you be happy, healthy, and live with ease.
May you be happy, healthy, and live with ease.
May you be happy, healthy, and live with ease.

Sending Loving-Kindness to Neutral People

Now think of someone you have held a grudge against, feel indifferent toward, or someone you don't know very well. Are the feelings you have serving you? Now imagine, you are standing in front of this person. You are alike in your wish to have a good life and desire to be happy. Send forgiveness, warmth and love to that person.

Send all your wishes for well-being to that person, repeating the following phrases, silently:
May you be happy, may you be healthy, may you live with ease.
May you be happy, may you be healthy, may you live with ease.
May you be happy, may you be healthy, may you live with ease.

Repeat as needed to send forgiveness, kindness, and love.

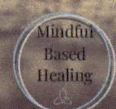

LOVING KINDNESS SCRIPT

Body Position
Close your eyes. Sit comfortably with your feet flat on the floor and your spine straight. Relax your whole body. Keep your eyes closed throughout the whole visualization and bring your awareness inward. Without straining or concentrating, just relax and gently follow the instructions.

Take a deep breath in. And breathe out.

Receiving Loving-Kindness
Keeping your eyes closed, think of a person close to you who loves you very much. It could be someone from the past or the present; someone still in life or who has transitioned; it could be a teacher or guide. Imagine that person standing in front of you, sending you their love. That person is sending you wishes for your safety, for your well-being and happiness. Feel the warm wishes, love or embrace coming from that person towards you.

Now bring to mind the same person or another person who cherishes you deeply. Imagine that person standing beside you, sending you wishes for your wellness, for your health and happiness. Feel the kindness and warmth coming to you from that person.

Now imagine that you are surrounded on all sides by all the people who love you and have loved you. Picture all of your friends and loved ones surrounding you, sending you wishes for your happiness, well-being, and health. Soak in the warmth, love and affection surrounding you. You are filled, and overflowing with warmth and love.

Today's thoughts

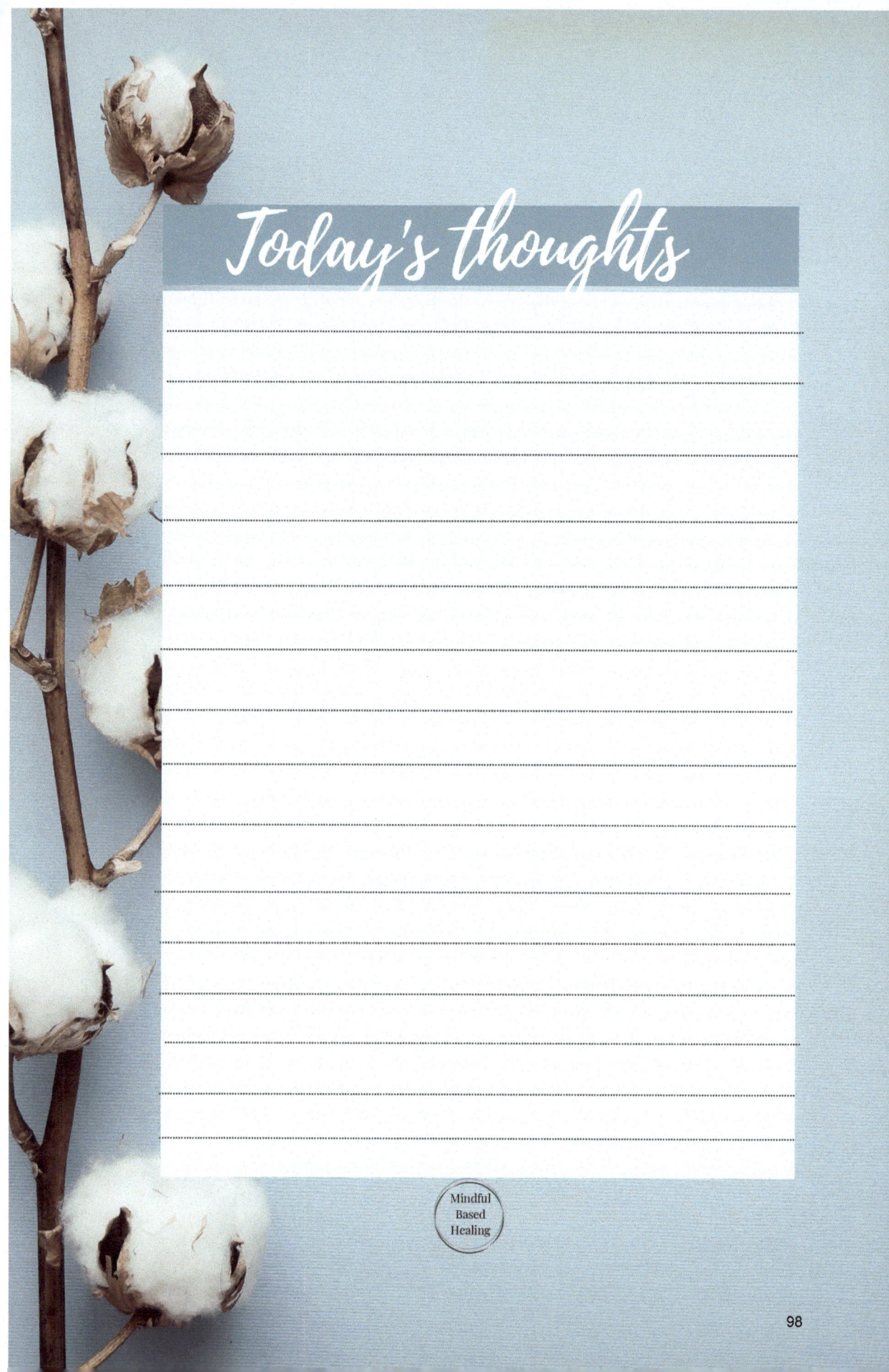

LOVING-KINDNESS

My experience with loving-kindness to others

My experience with loving-kindness to myself

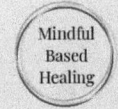

Today's thoughts

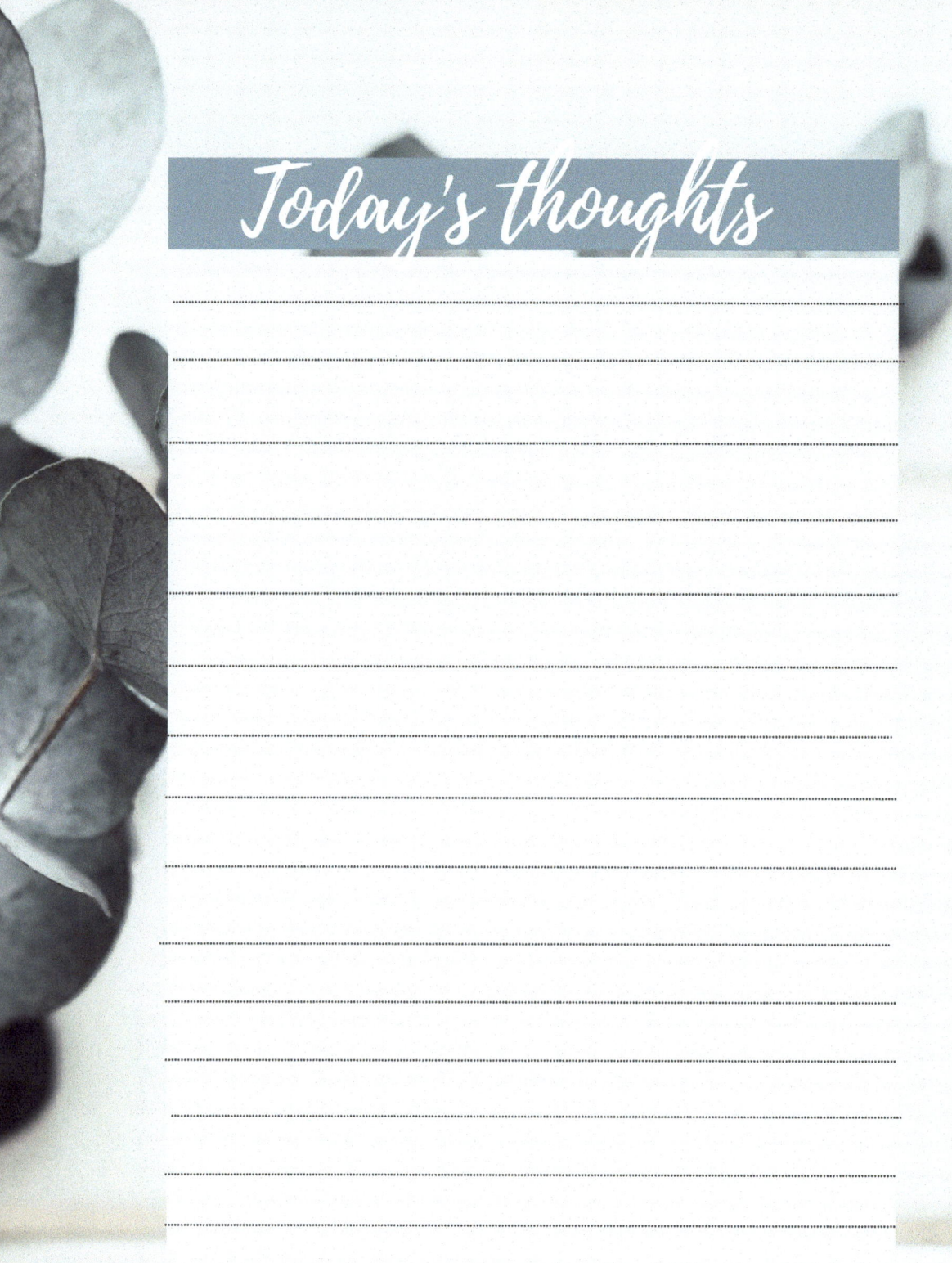

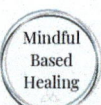

Mindful Based Healing

THE POWER OF FORGIVENESS

FORGIVE YOURSELF AND OTHERS

Think of someone who showed you love, kindness, forgiveness. How does it make you feel? Do you feel you deserve the affection? How does it impact your life?

Think of someone you may be holding a grudge against. How is that grudge making you feel? Is it supporting you or holding you back? What would it look like to let it go? Imagine forgiving that person or people. Imagine letting go of any negative feelings, thoughts, or emotions.
What does that feel like to you?

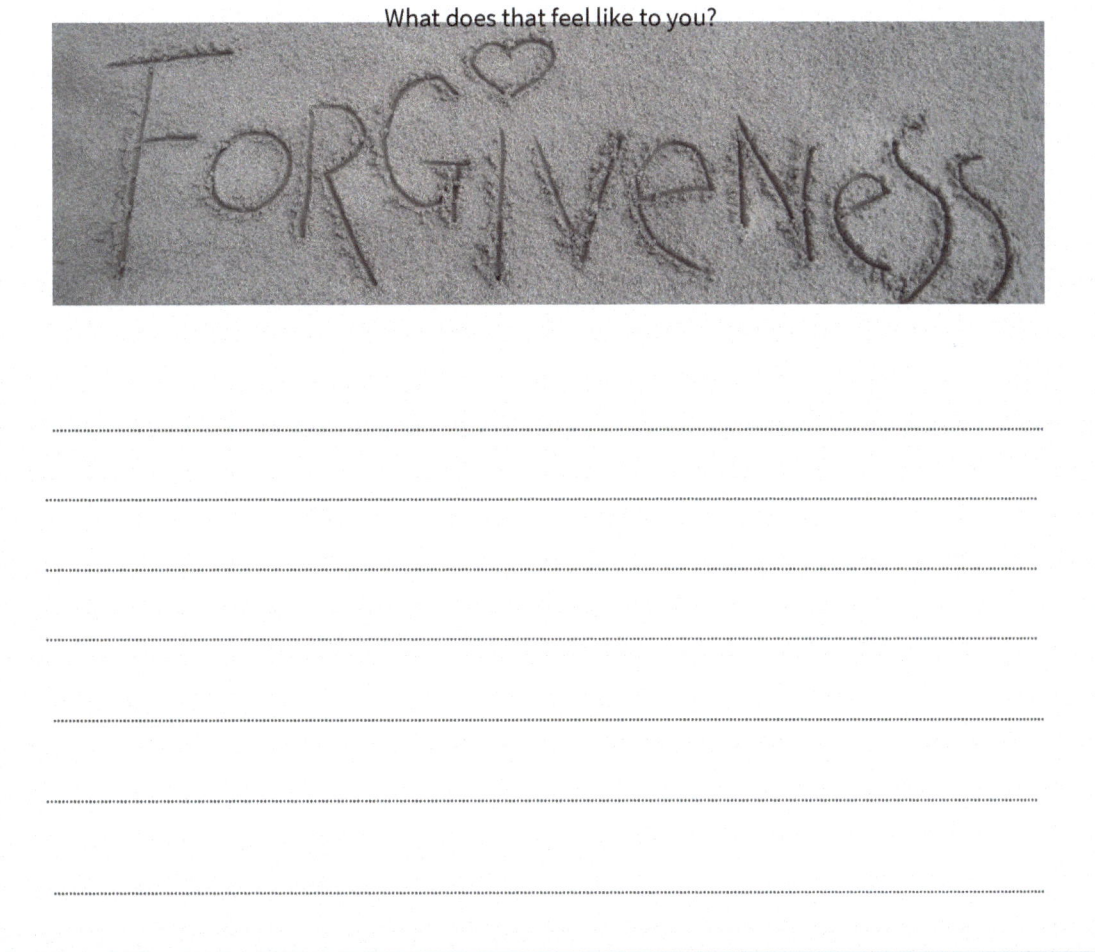

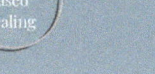

TODAY WAS GREAT BECAUSE

MY SELF CARE ACTIVITIES INCLUDE

Mindful Based Healing

Today's thoughts

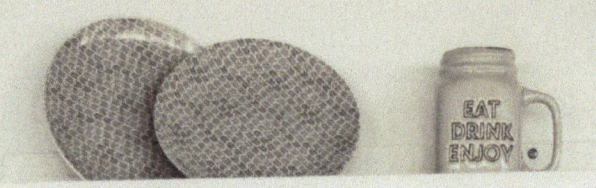

MINDFUL CONVERSATIONS

My experience with mindful listening

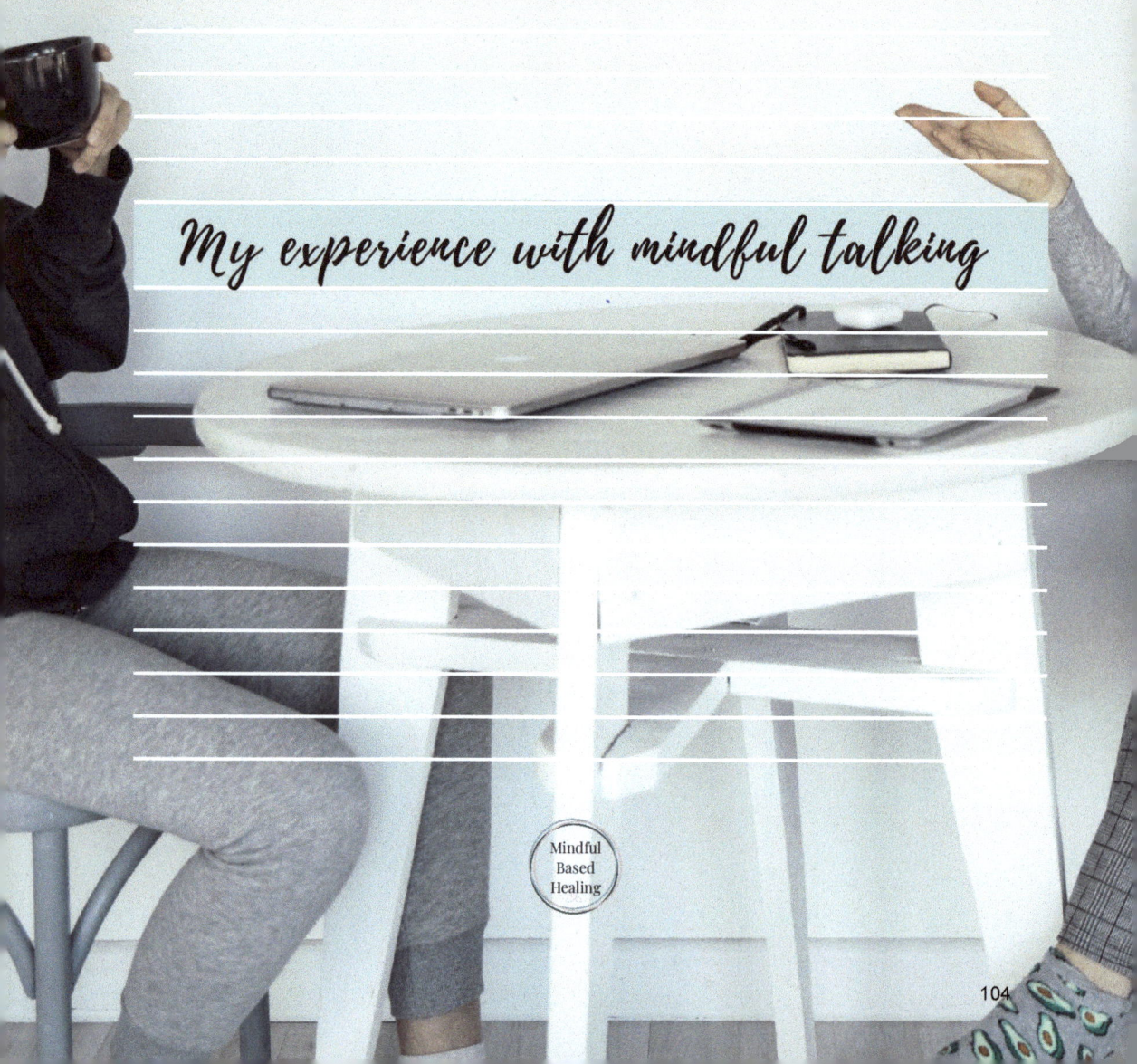

My experience with mindful talking

Today's thoughts

PART 7

MINDFUL COPING WITH SYMPTOMS AND EFFECTS OF TREATMENT

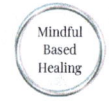

Acceptance

Coming to terms with things as they are. By denying or resisting what is (cancer diagnosis, being overweight, scars, etc) we are forcing situations to be as we wish, not as they are, which may lead to stress, anxiety, depression. This depletes our body from the energy to heal, accept, and progress to be made. For example, waiting to love yourself until you are at your goal weight or in remission, prevents you from ever loving or accepting yourself. It prevents you from enjoying your life or making progress toward your goal. Once you accept what is and love yourself anyway, the goal becomes less important and perhaps even easier.

Mindful Based Healing

Today's thoughts

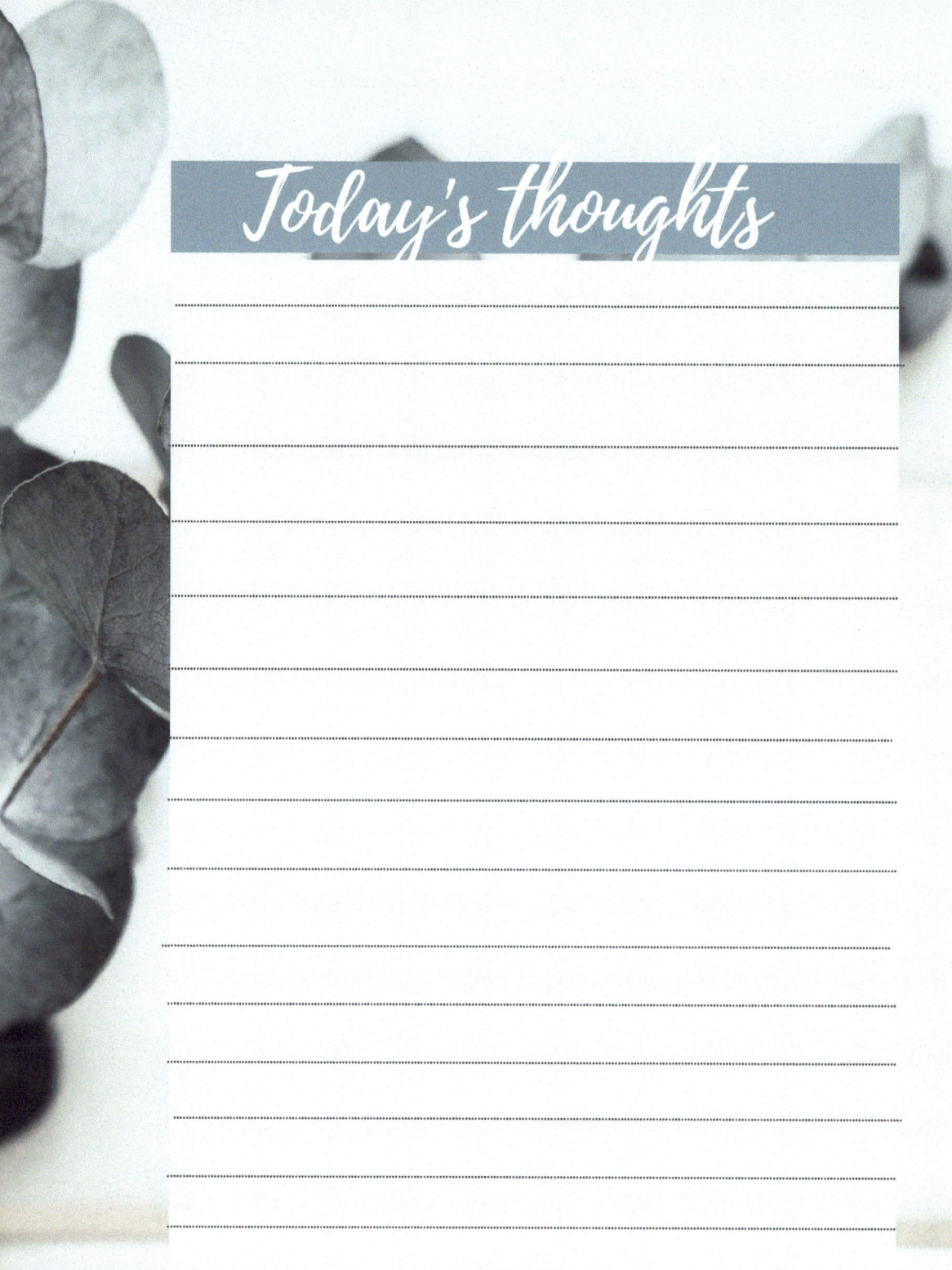

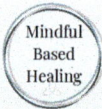

A TASTE OF MINDFULNESS

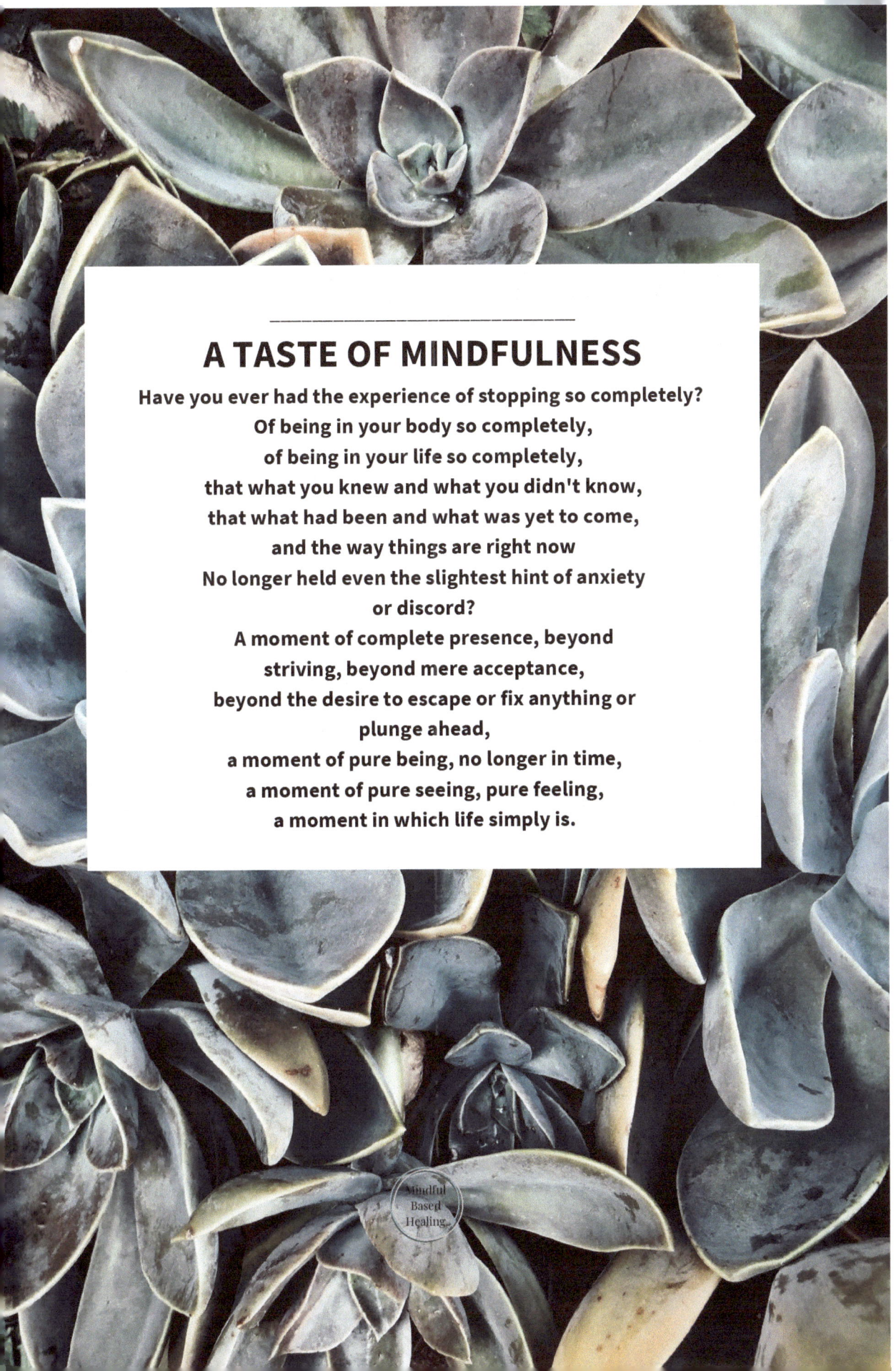

Have you ever had the experience of stopping so completely?
Of being in your body so completely,
of being in your life so completely,
that what you knew and what you didn't know,
that what had been and what was yet to come,
and the way things are right now
No longer held even the slightest hint of anxiety
or discord?
A moment of complete presence, beyond
striving, beyond mere acceptance,
beyond the desire to escape or fix anything or
plunge ahead,
a moment of pure being, no longer in time,
a moment of pure seeing, pure feeling,
a moment in which life simply is.

Today's thoughts

Mindful Based Healing

Today's thoughts

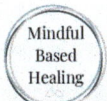

Self-Talk

How you speak to yourself has a direct impact on your health. Both positive and negative self-talk affects the left frontal and temporal regions of your brain.

Be patient, gentle, show love, speak kindly.

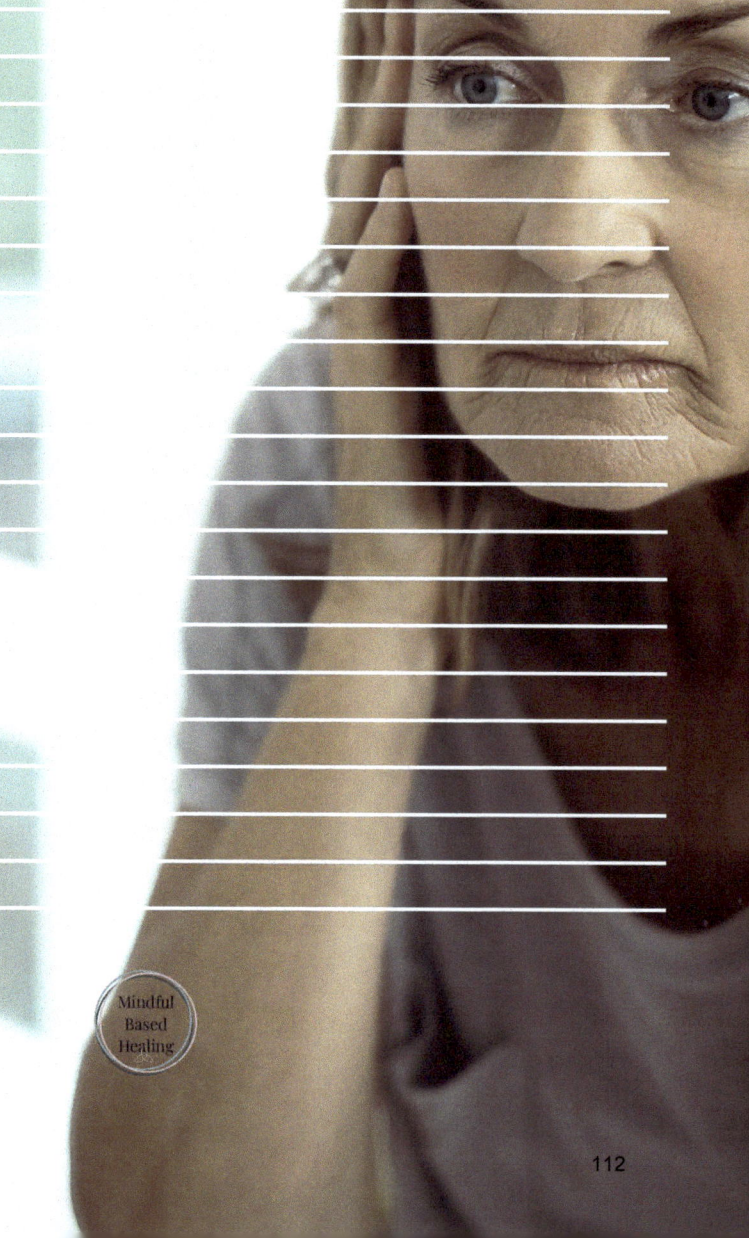

Today's thoughts

APPOINTMENT

Appointment date:_____

Help your healthcare providers give you the best care possible. Write down questions, take notes, and speak openly about your needs. If you need help or resources to follow the plan....ask!
They can't help you if you don't help yourself.

Concerns	Notes
	_____
	_____
	_____
	_____

Next steps	What support do I need to succeed?
_____	
_____	
_____	

Follow up

Mindful Based Healing

MY SIDE EFFECTS

DIAGNOSIS:

MENTAL:

DATE:

EMOTIONAL:

DATE:

PHYSICAL:

DATE:

HOW I SUPPORT MYSELF: **WHAT SUPPORT I NEED:**

Mindful Based Healing

Today's thoughts

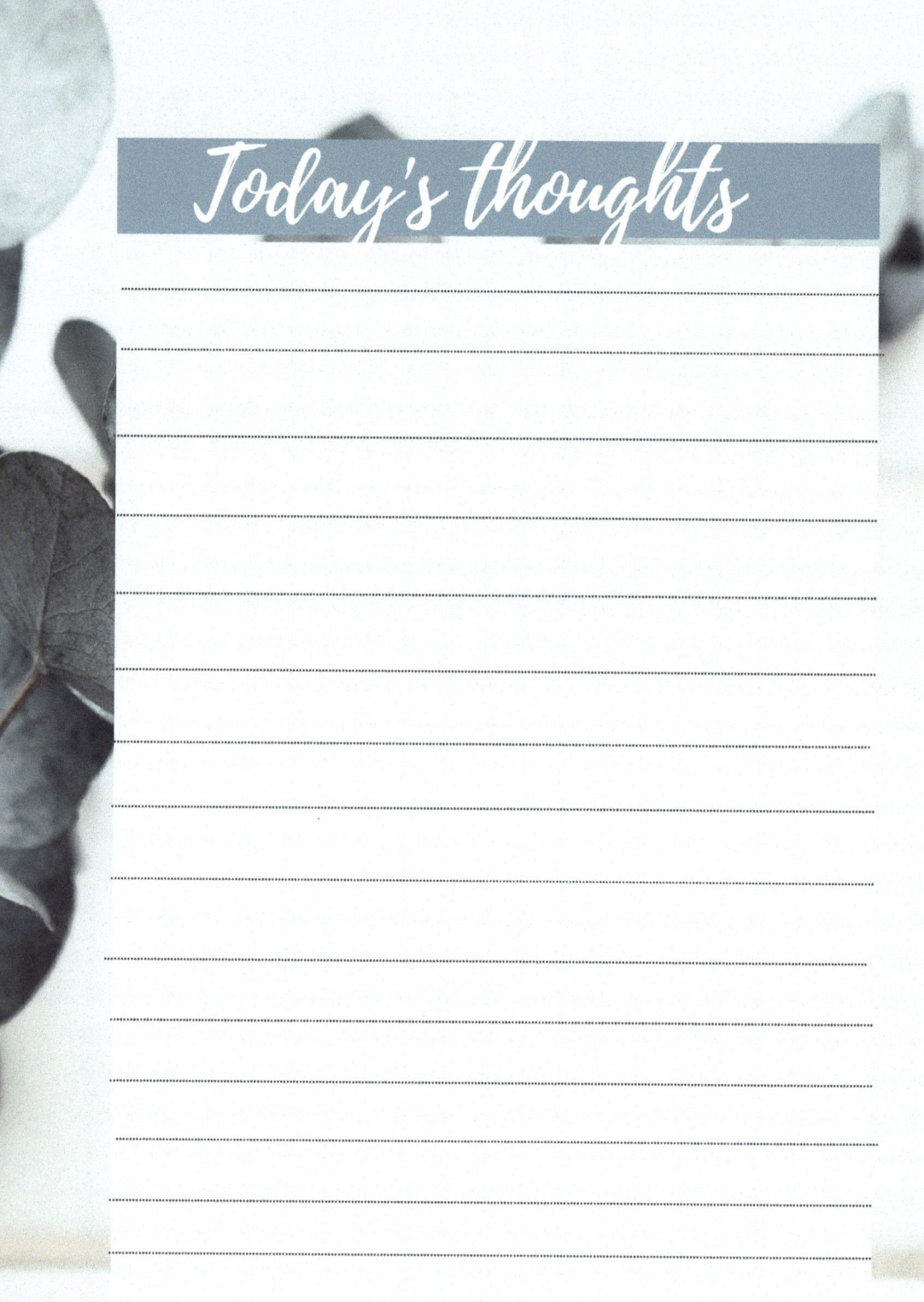

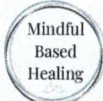

ADDRESSING FEARS

Often times it is not the fear itself, but the lack of control or knowing that makes one fear. Write down your fears and the actions you can take to prevent the fear from controlling you.
*Listen to associated audio for examples

Fear 1

Actions I can take:

Fear 2

Actions I can take:

Fear 3

Actions I can take:

Fear 4

Actions I can take:

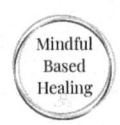

Today's thoughts

Mindful Based Healing

Heal from past trauma

What emotions or feelings make you uncomfortable? _____
What is it about that feeling that isn't pleasant? _____
Are you ashamed? _____
Do you allow yourself to feel and process these feelings or do you suppress?
_____
Why?_____
_____
_____
__

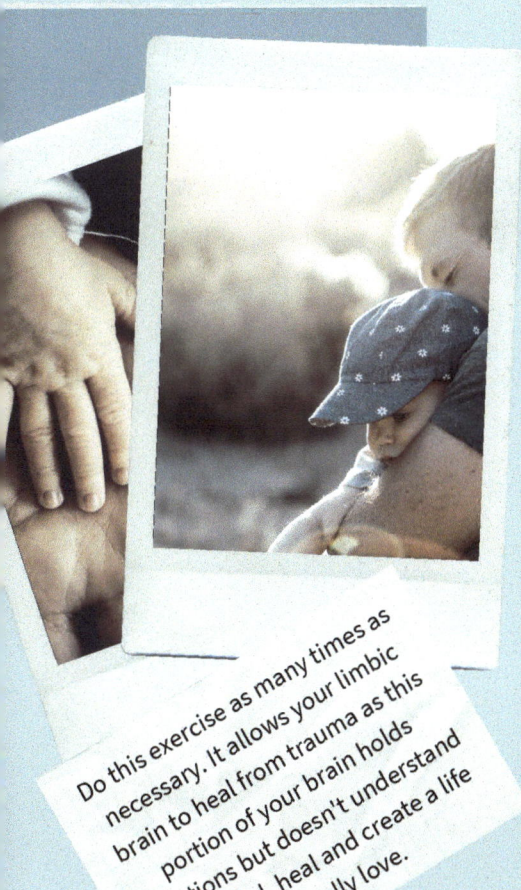

Close your eyes and imagine that feeling and the time of your life that it is most present.
How old are you? _____
What triggers that emotion?
_____

Now imagine in as much detail as possible the younger version of you as that feeling. Would you treat younger you as you do the emotion? Would you not allow younger you in the door or a seat at the table?
_____

Now give younger you a hug, attention, or words that you need to hear, feel, heal. Help that version of you know you are worthy, important, valued, loved, accepted, wanted.
_____
_____
_____

Do this exercise as many times as necessary. It allows your limbic brain to heal from trauma as this portion of your brain holds emotions but doesn't understand time. Feel, heal and create a life you really love.

Mindful Based Healing

Self- love
I am practicing self-love by:

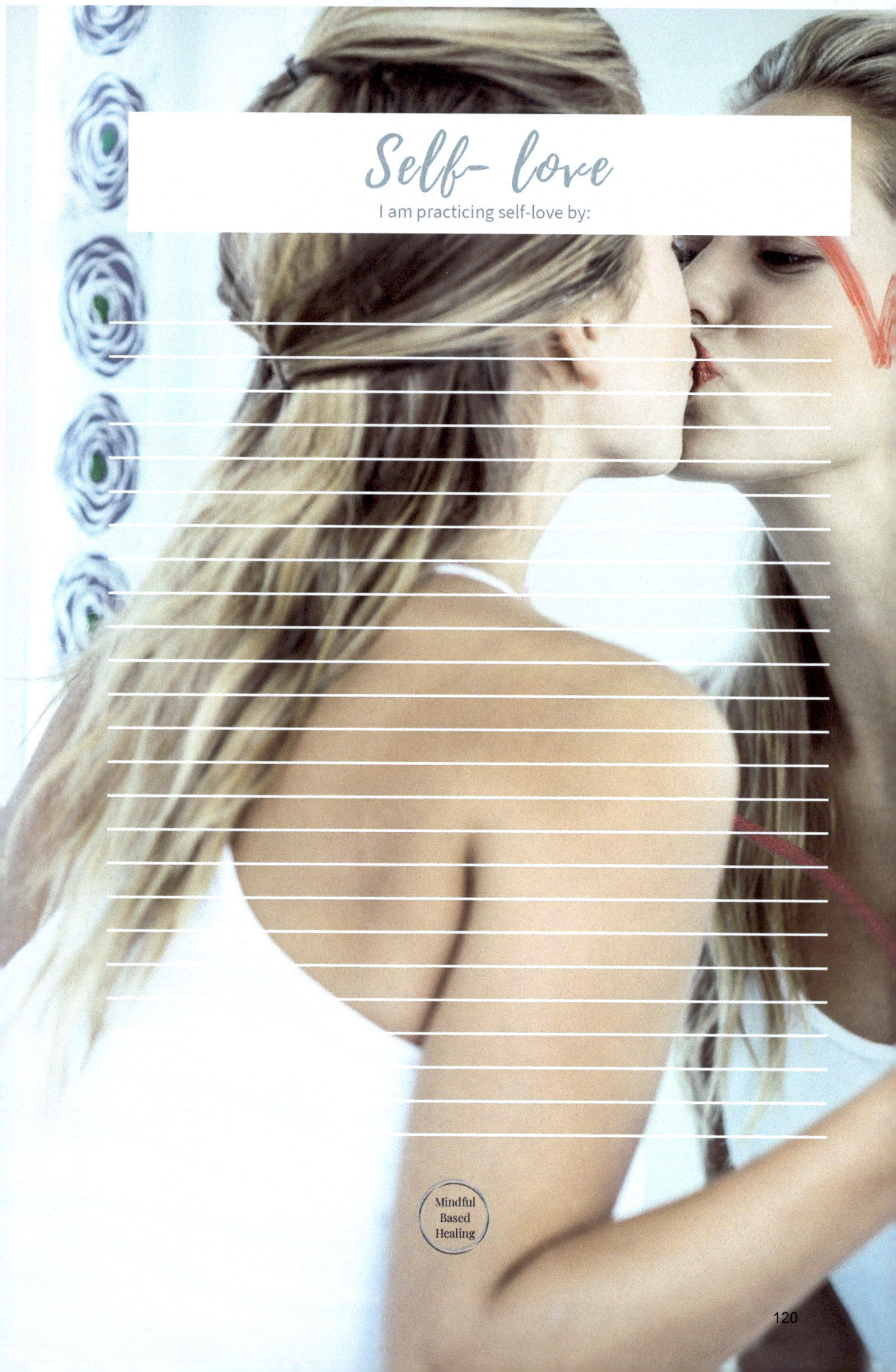

Today's thoughts

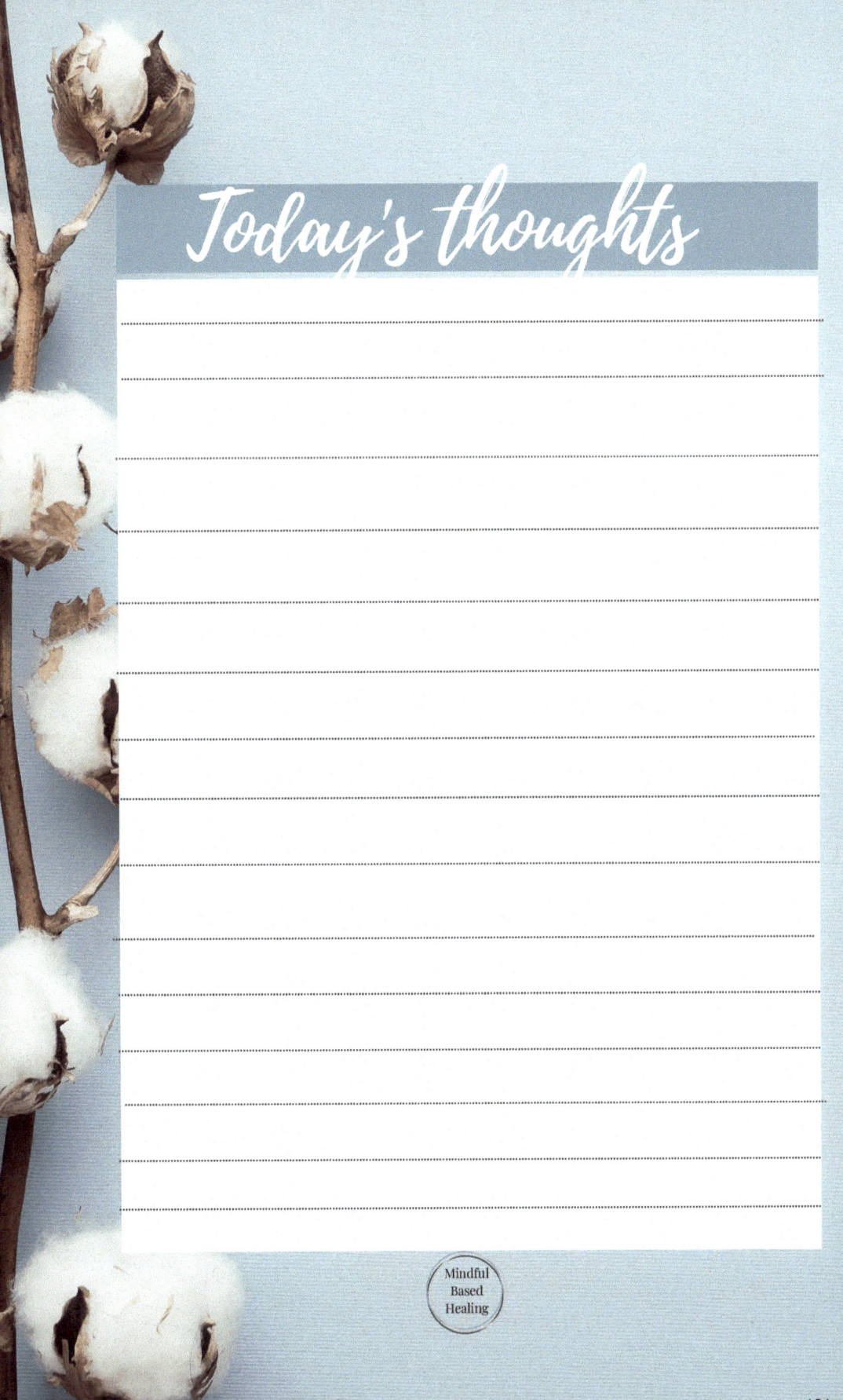

SELF-CARE TRACKER

ACTIVITY: S M T W T F S

NOTES: _____

Today's thoughts

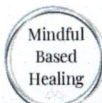

MINDFUL BODY TRACKER

As you begin to be more present, you may be more aware of how food, medication or activity affects your body. Take note on how you are fueling and supporting your body during this time.

✓ When I (eat/ drink/ move/ take):	My body feels:

Notes

Today's thoughts

Mindful Based Healing

PART 8

MEDITATION STYLES

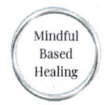

DEVELOPING A PERSONAL PRACTICE

1. Choose how you want to live your life.
2. In order to live life fully, be present for it with awareness to the moments.
3. Pay attention on purpose, in the moment, without judgment.
4. Practice loving-kindness toward yourself and others.
5. Experiencing good /bad, pleasant /unpleasant, in the moment is the time to learn, grow, see what is really going on, – even in the face of pain and suffering.
6. Focus on "being" rather than "doing".
7. Find mindfulness and meditative style that resonates with you.
8. You are not your thoughts, opinions, likes or dislikes. They are thought bubbles and you don't have to be imprisoned by them.
9. This is hard, it takes practice, and it's worth it.
10. Decide how long to *try* practicing and stick with it.

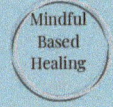

Mindful Based Healing

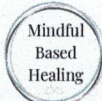

Today's thoughts

Mindful Based Healing

Today's thoughts

Mindful Based Healing

MANTRA AS AN ANCHOR

*Seek appropriate support if you experience feelings of overwhelm.

A mantra (mind-vehicle) is a powerful tool and can be used to help ground you in awareness. Much like focusing on your breath, a mantra can be used to gently bring you back to the present when you notice thoughts taking control or easily distracted. Use with gentleness and ease, silently reciting, like a feather lightly brushing your cheek.

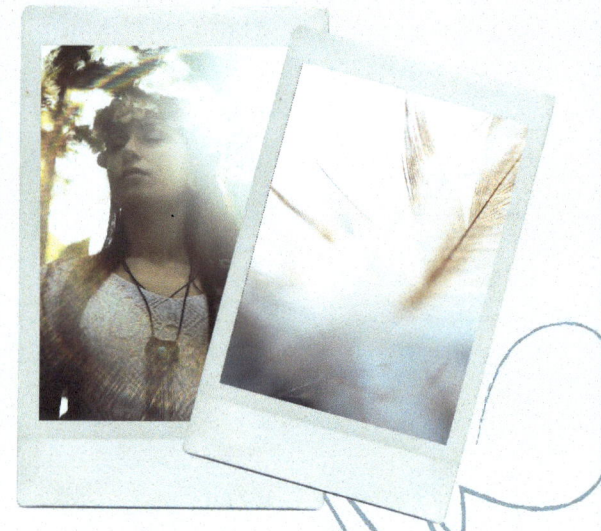

According to Dharma Sing Khalsa, M.D, "Mantras stimulate the secretions of the pituitary gland...certain permutations send signals to the command centers of the brain —the hypothalamus, and the pituitary... [which] orchestrate a healing response and send out packets of information in the form of neurotransmitters and chemicals, in the brain and throughout the body."

Sample Mantras:
- Om (Aum) or One : unity
- Satya (SAHTH-yah): truth
- Prana (PRAH-na): life force
- Prajna (PRUHG-nah): wisdom
- Niyama (NEEYA-mah): observance

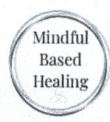

Mindful Based Healing

Today's thoughts

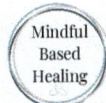

MEDITATION AND MINDFULNESS

There are numerous meditation and mindfulness techniques. I have simplified them into four categories to help facilitate the learning and benefits. Try out various types and duration to find the best fit for you. Empower yourself to heal, enjoy life, and be your own advocate.
Each type begins with breath and body scan as the foundation.

1 **Focused meditation-** focus on breath and/ or body sensations while doing body scan. (5-45 minutes daily)

2 **Mantra or anchor meditation-** use a mantra, word or phrase as the anchor for being present and allow breath to flow freely. Allow the last few minutes free of focus, in gratitude or silence. Begin with 5-10 minutes daily, work toward 15 minutes, twice per day.

3 **Loving-kindness meditation-** direct feelings of love and compassion to yourself and others to cultivate compassion. It's a great way to let go of negativity and improve your overall mood. Option to massage body during body scan. (5-45 minutes daily)

4 **Guided meditation-** Guided journey with instructor's words, imagery or sound. (10-45 minutes daily) Find guided meditations at: **mindfulbasedhealing.com/meditation**

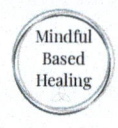

Mindful Based Healing

Today's thoughts

7 MYTHS OF MEDITATION

In the past 40 years, meditation has entered the mainstream of modern Western culture; its been prescribed by physicians and practiced by everyone from business executives, artists, and scientists to students, teachers, military personnel. Despite the growing popularity of meditation, misconceptions still prevent many people from trying meditation and receiving its healing benefits for the body, mind, and spirit.

Myth #1: Meditation is difficult.

Truth: This myth is rooted in the perception that meditation is reserved for saints, holy people, or spiritual adepts. In reality, with clear instruction from an experienced teacher, meditation can be easy and fun to learn. Techniques can be as simple as focusing on the breath or silently repeating a mantra. Meditation may seem difficult if we try too hard to concentrate, are overly attached to results, or worry if we are doing it right.

Myth #2: Clear your mind to have a successful meditation practice.

Truth: This is one of the most common misconceptions which causes many people to give up in frustration. Meditation isn't about stopping thoughts or clearing the mind -- both of these approaches create stress and discourage trying or continuing a meditative practice. Thoughts can not be stopped, but we can decide how much attention to give them. Through meditation we can find the quiet that already exists in the space *between* our thoughts. This space allows pure consciousness, pure silence, and pure peace.

In meditation, the use of a metaphoric anchor, such as breath, an image, or a mantra, allows the mind to relax into a silent stream of awareness. When thoughts arise, as they inevitably will, don't judge or push them away. Instead, gently return attention to your anchor. In every meditation, there are moments when the mind dips and experiences pure awareness. The more consistent the practice, the more time in this state of expanded awareness and silence will be experienced.

Even if it feels like thoughts have been consistent and dominant throughout the meditation, time has not been wasted. Awareness of these thoughts is success.

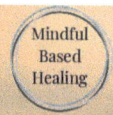

Mindful Based Healing

Myth #3: It takes years of dedicated practice to receive any benefits from meditation.
Truth: Benefits can be experienced in the first meditation and will be more cumulative and profound with the consistency of a regular practice. Many scientific studies, such as the one led by Harvard University and Massachusetts General Hospital, provide evidence of profound affects including decreased anxiety, greater feelings of calm, growth in the areas of the brain associated with memory, empathy, sense of self, and stress regulation, within just eight weeks of practice.

Myth #4: Meditation is escapism.
Truth: The purpose of meditation isn't to tune out or get away; rather tune in and get in touch with your true self. Meditation allows one to go below the mind's churning, which tends to be filled with repetitive thoughts about the past and worries about the future, into the still point of pure consciousness. In this state, one is able let go of the stories, limiting beliefs, and stress.

As the practice becomes more regular, the window of perception cleanses and clarity expands. There are a variety of meditation techniques, find one that works for you. Also consider working with a therapist who can help you safely explore and heal from past pain or trauma, especially if emotions get too intense.

Myth #5: I don't have enough time to meditate.
Truth: There are busy, productive executives who have not missed a meditation in 25 years. Even a few minutes of meditation is better than none.
With a regular meditation practice, one is able to experience the fourth state of consciousness ,in which there is greater ability to accomplish more by doing less. In this restful state, there is alertness that is extremely refreshing for the body and mind. Instead of struggling to achieve goals, there is more time spent "in the flow" which allows for more clear and creative thinking.

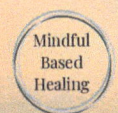

Mindful Based Healing

Myth #6: Meditation requires spiritual or religious beliefs.
Truth: Meditation is a practice for beyond the noisy chatter of the mind into stillness and silence. It doesn't require a specific spiritual belief, and people of many different religions practice meditation without any conflict with their religious beliefs. Meditate in order to experience inner quiet and the physical, mental and emotional health benefits; including enhanced concentration, lowered blood pressure, stress reduction, stronger immune system and more restful sleep. Meditation enables one to enjoy life more fully and happily.

Myth #7: I'm supposed to have transcendent experiences in meditation.
Truth: Some people are disappointed when they don't experience visions, see colors, levitate, hear a choir of angels, or glimpse enlightenment during meditation. Although there are wonderful experiences, including feelings of bliss and oneness, this isn't the purpose. The real benefits of meditation are what happens in the other hours of the day, as some of the stillness and silence of the practice carry forward, allowing for more creativity, compassion, and loving-kindness to ourselves and others.

_____

As you begin or continue your meditation journey, here are some other guidelines that may help you on your way:

1. No expectations. Sometimes the mind is too active to settle down, or it settles down immediately. Be gentle and let go of expectations.
2. Give yourself grace. Meditation isn't about getting it *right* or *wrong*. It's about awareness, then letting your mind find its true awareness.
3. Find a meditation technique that resonates with you. There are many types of meditations, try a few and use the one(s) that feel best for you.
4. Unplug. Try to ensure no one and nothing will disturb you.
5. Come with the intent to meditate. If your attention is somewhere else; you won't find silence. Your intention must be clear and free of other obligations.

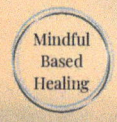

Today's thoughts

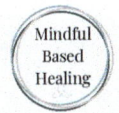

Mindful Based Healing

UNCONDITIONAL

Willing to experience aloneness,
I discover connection everywhere;
Turning to face my fear,
I meet the warrior who lives within;
Opening to my loss,
I gain the embrace of the universe;
Surrendering into emptiness,
I find fullness without end.

Each condition I flee from pursues me,
Each condition I welcome transforms me
And becomes itself transformed
Into its radiant jewel-like essence.
I bow to the one who has made it so,
Who has crafted this Master Game;
To play it is purest delight;
To honor its form – true devotion.

© Jennifer Welwood

Today's thoughts

Mindful Based Healing

CURRENT STRUGGLES

....

....

....

....

....

HOW I CAN ASK FOR SUPPORT

....

....

....

....

....

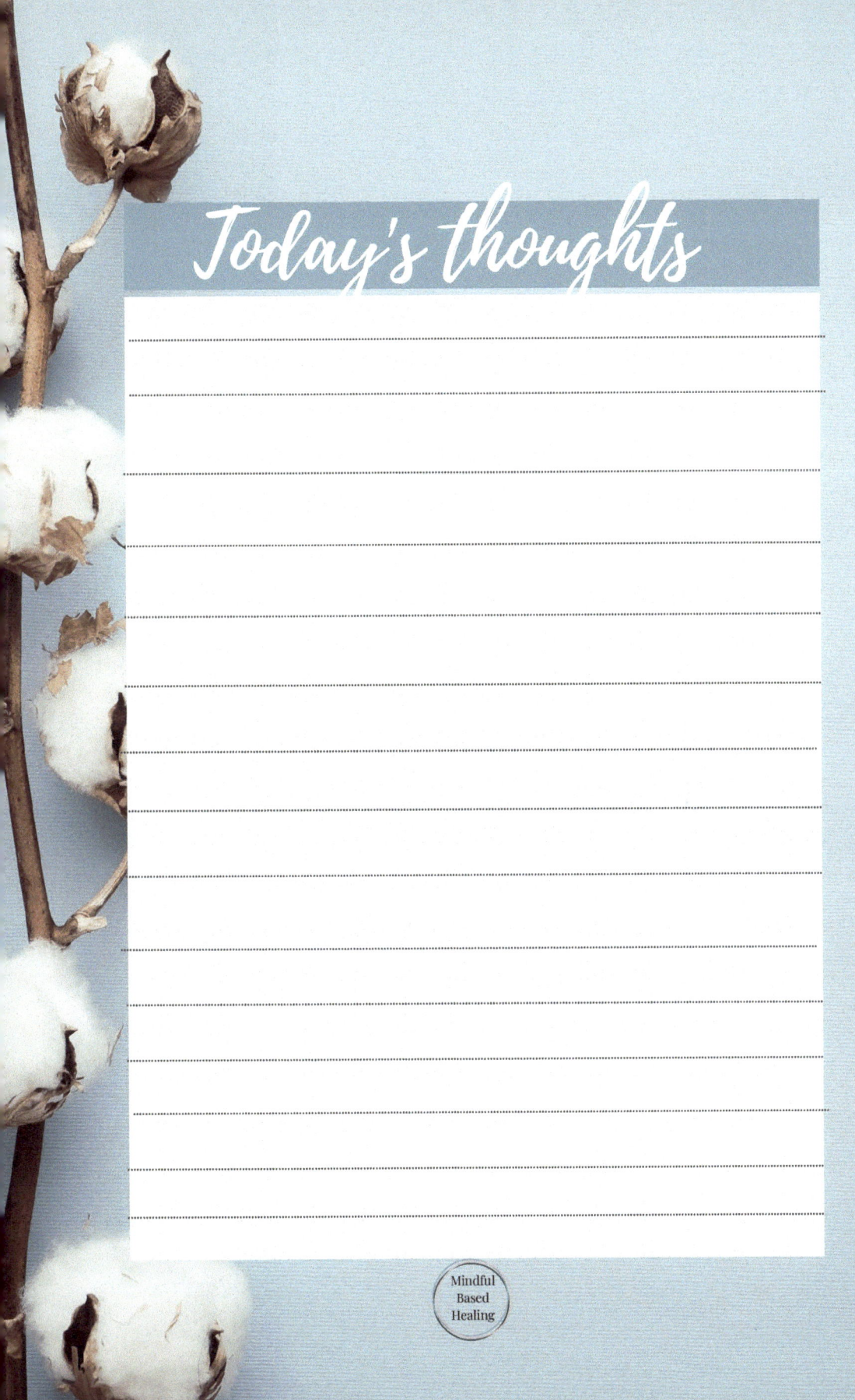

Today's thoughts

Mindful Based Healing

PART 9

BEYOND TREATMENT, FINDING YOUR NEW NORMAL

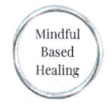

Non-striving

Often we perform action with intent to accomplish something. In life, can you think of anything you've been striving for or working toward? What was the result? Did you cause you stress during the process? Did it make you tense? It's healthy to identify goals, but in the mindfulness practice, the goal is not striving to reach them. Allow them to unfold throughout the experience.

Today's thoughts

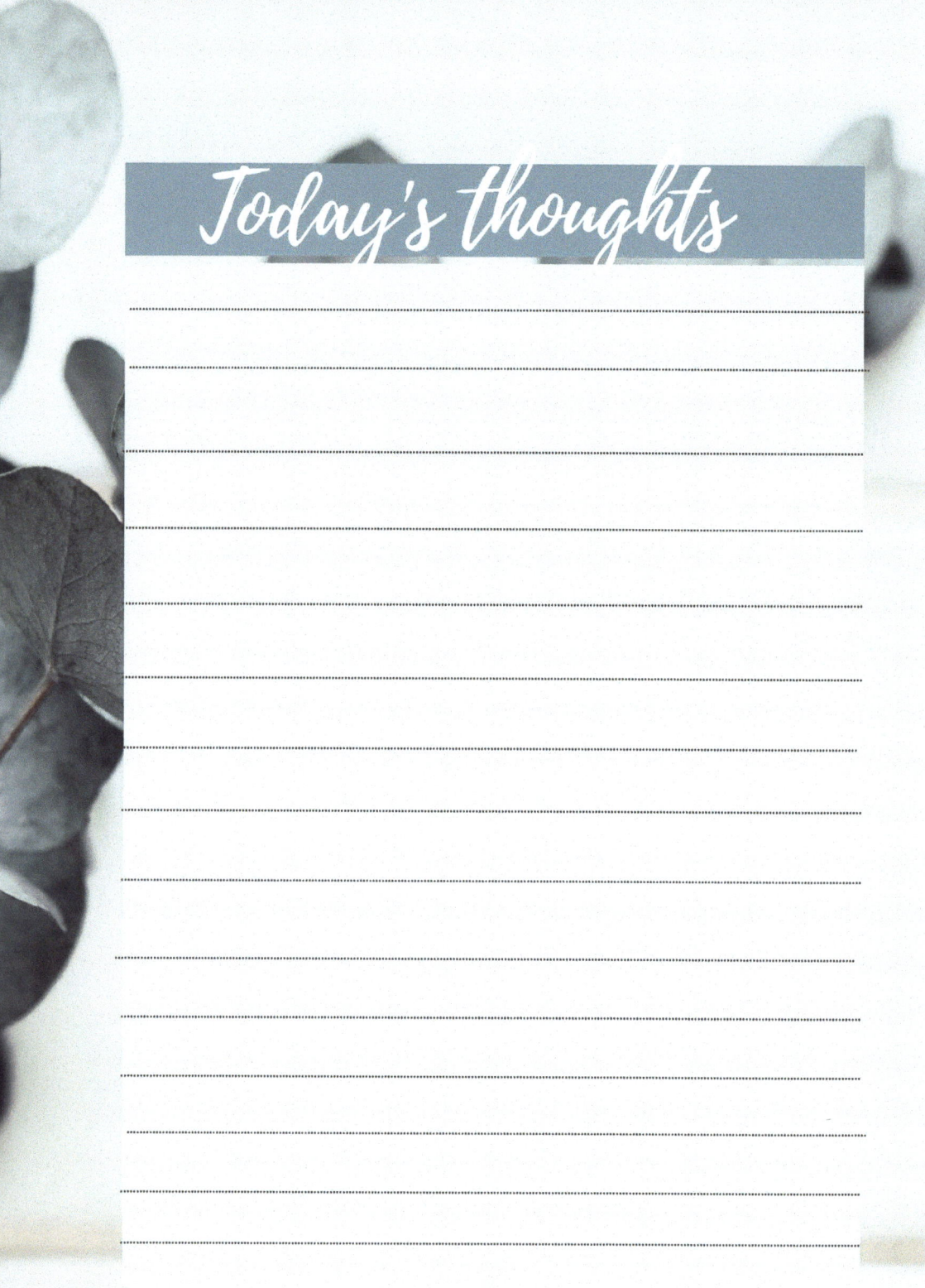

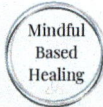

NEXT STEPS

Now that treatments have concluded and it's time to find your new normal; you may feel a bit lost, anxious or uncertain. You have the tools to be present, the resilience to create a life that aligns with what is important to you, and the ability to no longer be controlled by thoughts or worry.

Take action. Focus on what is most important to you.

Be proactive. Speak with your boss about flexible hours or working from home.

Be prepared. Write down what you want and how it supports you and your company to get the flexibility you are requesting.

Ask for help! Get continued support from family and friends while you readjust to this new routine.

Give back. Volunteer, propose a wellness workshop at your workplace or donate for others to experience the healing powers of mindfulness.

For more information visit:
MindfulBasedHealing.com/courses or
MindfulBasedHealing.com/donate

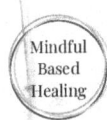

Mindful Based Healing

PRIORITIES

It is easy to get caught up in the hustle, bustle and expectations of life. Quality of life is not measured by the quantity of time, but rather on how time is spent. What are your priorities? Do your actions reflect this? *(Hint: assess your priorities, then schedule them in your calendar to help you stay focused)*

PRIORITY:	HOW AM I SUPPORTING PRIORITY:
PRIORITY:	HOW AM I SUPPORTING PRIORITY:
PRIORITY:	HOW AM I SUPPORTING PRIORITY:

Mindful Based Healing

Today's thoughts

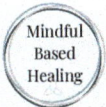

SELF-REFLECTION

You are not the same as when you started. Take a moment to acknowledge how far you've come.

○ What has this journey taught you?

○ How do you feel?

○ How are you different?

○ What have you learned?

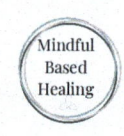

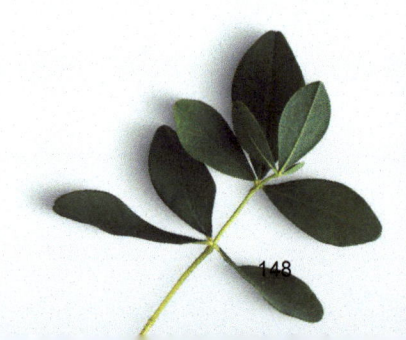

Mindful Based Healing

Today's thoughts

THE 'NEW' YOU
Visualize the life you want
BE SPECIFIC AND TAKE ACTION

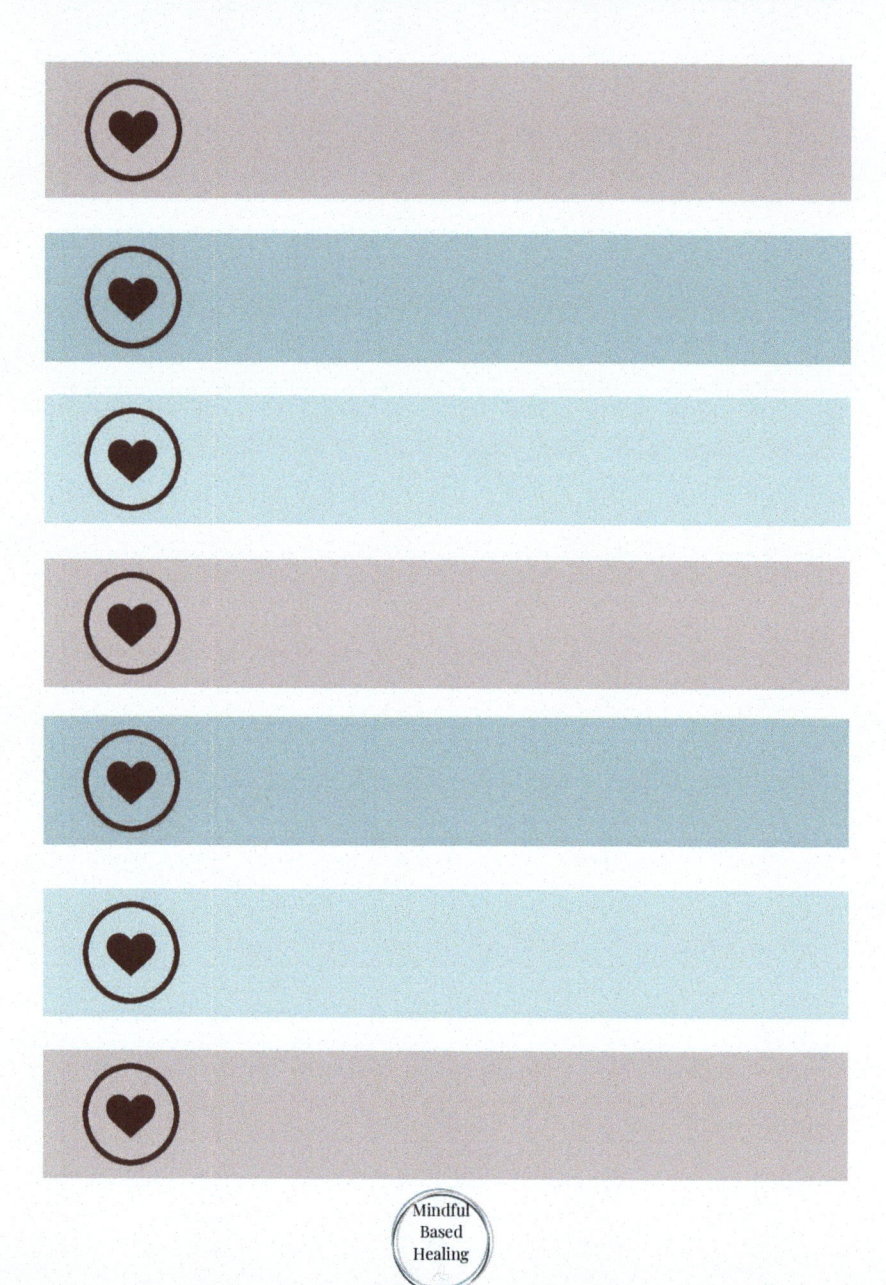

- ♥
- ♥
- ♥
- ♥
- ♥
- ♥
- ♥

Mindful Based Healing

Today's thoughts

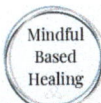

Mindful Based Healing

SELF-CARE TRACKER

ACTIVITY: S M T W T F S

NOTES: _____

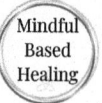

MORNING CHECKLIST

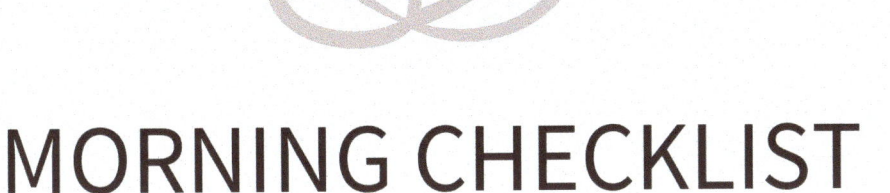

SCHEDULE YOUR DAY FOR SUCCESS

- ☐ make your bed
- ☐ brush teeth & wash face
- ☐ meditation or journal
- ☐ mindful movement
- ☐ healthy food to fuel your body

Enjoy your day!

Today's thoughts

THIRTY DAYS OF KINDNESS

Small actions can lead to big impact. Use this challenge as inspiration to be kind to yourself or others. Be creative and come up with your own ideas. I encourage you to document your experience. How did it feel to show appreciation or an act of kindness? Did it give you fulfillment?

1 Talk a walk outside	2 Journal	3 Smile at a stranger	4 Sit quietly for 5 minutes	5 Take a bath
6 Color or draw	7 Eat your favorite dessert	8 Give a hug	9 Read a book or poem	10 Write 3 things you like most about yourself
11 Listen to your favorite song	12 Get a massage	13 Do yoga or gentle movement	14 Have coffee with a friend	15 Cook your favorite meal
16 Stop to smell some flowers	17 Ask for a hug	18 Write someone an appreciation note	19 Do a self-love massage	20 Say hi to a stranger
21 Forgive someone or yourself	22 Write yourself an appreciation note	23 Take a nap	24 Sing in the shower or car	25 Buy yourself flowers
26 Listen to an audio book	27 Say what you like about yourself out loud	28 Enjoy fresh air	29 Forgive someone	30 Love yourself

Mindful Based Healing

Today's thoughts

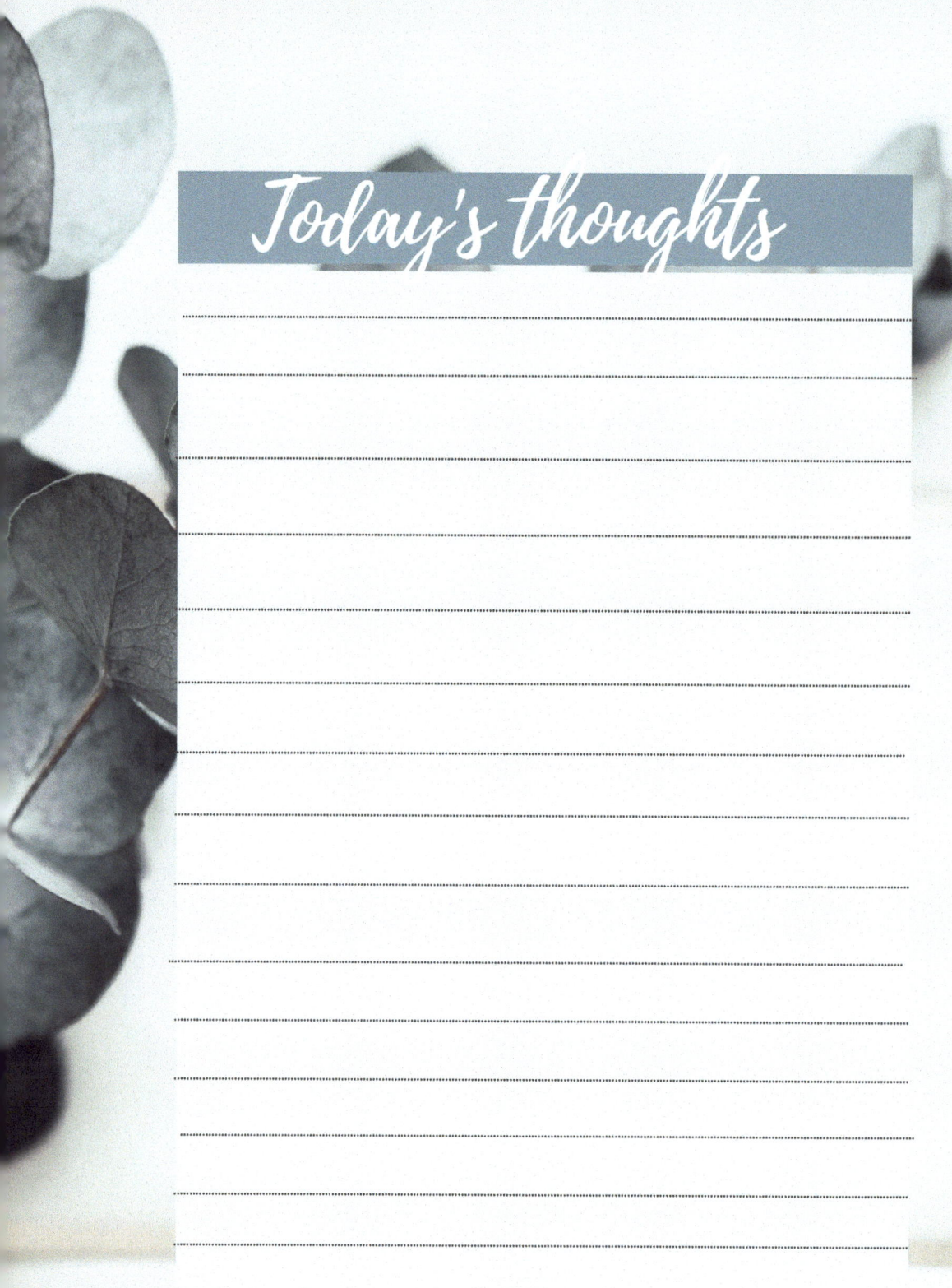

Today's thoughts

Mindful Based Healing

SELF ASSESSMENT
POST MINDFUL BASED HEALING

TODAY'S DATE

CATEGORIES
Please scale the following from 1-5
1 being excellent, 5 being poor.

Excellent-1   2   3   4   Poor-5

How would you rate your overall health?

How well have you been sleeping?

How is your mental and emotional health?

How is your anxiety level?

How is your current ability to cope with pain?

How much do you fully enjoy life?

Since starting this program, are you happier?

Yes   No   Unsure

NOTES

SCALE

1 = Excellent

2 = Very good

3 = Acceptable

4 = Having difficulty

5 = Poor

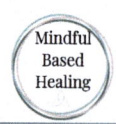

Mindful Based Healing

REAL PATIENT STORIES

These are real stories of patients who have made an impact on me over the years. I hope their stories inspire you as they have me.

*Not photos of actual patients in order to protect privacy.

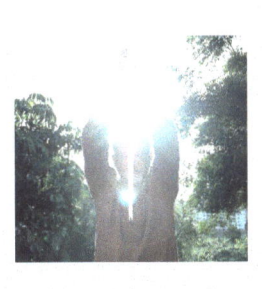

R.G.

'I am a very fortunate man. I fully understand these are my bonus days. I was diagnosed with stage IV non-small cell lung carcinoma and "failed out of the study" that could buy me some time. I wasn't supposed to be alive today. EACH DAY IS A GIFT. Thank you for your beautiful challenge. You are a beautiful person.' - Ron

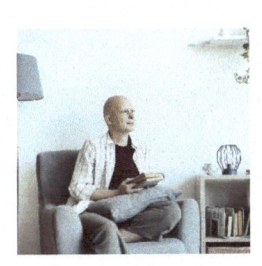

MARY

Mary was diagnosed with stage IV Glioblastoma multiform, an aggressive form of brain cancer. The typlcal outlook for this type of cancer is less than six months. Despite her diagnosis, Mary came to treatment everyday with a smile on her face. She was so inspiring to me. How can she be so happy when she's dying? Mary shared her secret with me. "We will all die one day honey, but that doesn't mean we have to be miserable until it happens. Heck, I could get hit by a bus on my way out of here." Mary finished her treatments and to my surprise, I saw her at her one year follow up! Mary's attitude and being present in the moment allowed her to *enjoy* her life, regardless of how long.

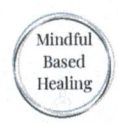

Mindful Based Healing

YOU DID IT!

Congratulations on completing this workbook! You can come back to the exercises anytime. Take a moment to acknowledge how far you have come. You are not the same person who started this journey, and I believe you will continue to evolve beyond. Prioritizing your health, learning to be present, and empowering yourself to be your own advocate is not an easy task. Keep going.

"Be thankful for what you are now and keep fighting for what you want to be tomorrow." - HERMI

I would *love* your feedback of the Mindful Based Healing journey. Feel free to reach out and share at:
hello@mindfuloncology.com

If you would like to continue your healing journey, please visit: **MindfulBasedHealing.com**

If you would like to donate for others to experience the benefits of this program, please visit:
MindfulBasedHealing.com/donate

MINDFULBASEDHEALING.COM

Mindful Based Healing

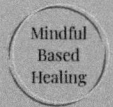

PART 10

INSPIRATION AND RESOURCES

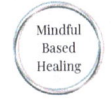

Mindful Based Healing

REFERENCES

This publication is designed to provide accurate and authoritative information in regard to the subject matter covered. It is sold with the understanding that the author is not engaged in rendering psychological, financial, legal or other professional services. If expert assistance or counseling is needed, the services of a competent professional should be sought.

THE ART OF COMMUNICATING by Thich Nhat Hanh, copyright ©2014 by Harper Collins Publishers.

PERFECT HEALTH by Deepak Chopra, copyright ©2000 by Deepak Chopra.

MBSR, Mindfulness Based Stress Reduction by Jon Kabat-Zinn provided by Mindful Leader.

CLINICIANS GUIDE TO TEACHING MINDFULNESS by Christiane Wolf and J. Greg Serpa, copyright ©2015 by Christiane Wolf and J. Greg Serpa.

FULL CATASTROPHE LIVING by Jon Kabat-Zinn, copyright ©1990 by Jon Kabat-Zinn.

"Love after Love" from COLLECTED POEMS 1948-1984 by Derek Walcott. Copyright ©1986 by Derek Walcott.

Elizabeth Scott. (2020, August 3). *What Is Stress?* https://www.verywellmind.com/stress-and-health-3145086

Alvin Powell. (2018, April 9). *When Science Meets Mindfulness.* The Harvard Gazette. https://news.harvard.edu/gazette/story/2018/04/harvard-researchers-study-how-mindfulness-may-change-the-brain-in-depressed-patients/

Jeena Cho. (2016, July 14). *Six Scientifically Proven Benefits of Mindfulness and Meditation.* Forbes. https://www.forbes.com/sites/jeenacho/2016/07/14/10-scientifically-proven-benefits-of-mindfulness-and-meditation/?sh=58beaaae63ce

Linda E. Carlson, Michael Speca, Peter Faris, Kamala D. Patel. (2007). *One year pre–post intervention follow-up of psychological, immune, endocrine and blood pressure outcomes of mindfulness-based stress reduction (MBSR) in breast and prostate cancer outpatients.* Brain, Behavior, and Immunity, Volume 21, Issue 8. https://www.sciencedirect.com/science/article/abs/pii/S0889159107000852.

Jill Suttie. (2018, October 29). *5 Science-Backed Reasons Mindfulness Meditation Is Good for Your Health.* https://www.mindful.org/five-ways-mindfulness-meditation-is-good-for-your-health.

STUFF I LOVE

These are items I personally love and/ or I have heard from former cancer fighters, which supported their journeys. I have no affiliation or compensation from any of these companies at the time this book is being produced.

- Aquaphor skin cream- My family and I use this on everything. During treatment useee for after radiation treatments, cuts, or rough skin. **www.aquaphorus.com**
- Ginger candies for nausea
- Nail strengthener to protect nails during chemotherapy treatment
- Aloe Gloe drinks for head and neck patients so hydrate and soothe the throat (*This brand is delicious, some others are not)* **www.gloebrands.com**
- Suja cold pressed juice- Ubers greens is my favorite and it helped me stop takingee over 30+ pills per day and get my health back on track **www.sujajuice.com**
- *Braving The Wilderness* and *The Gifts of Imperfection* by Brene Brown
- *Perfect Health* by Deepak Chopra, MD

SONGS TO FUEL YOUR FIGHT

- Here Comes The Sun by The Beatles
- Fight Song by Rachel Platten
- Good Life by One Republic
- Better When I'm Dancing by Meghan Trainor
- Happy by Pharrell
- Ceiling Can't Hold Us by Mackelmore
- Brave by Sarah Bareilles
- Best Day Of My Life by American Authors
- Dancing Queen by ABBA